God's Design for the

Highly Healthy Person

Formerly titled *10 Essentials of Highly Healthy People*

Walt Larimore, M.D.

WITH TRACI MULLINS

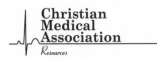

Christian
Medical
Association
Resources

ZONDERVAN™

GRAND RAPIDS, MICHIGAN 49530 USA

We want to hear from you. Please send your comments about this book to us in care of zreview@zondervan.com. Thank you.

ZONDERVAN™

God's Design for the Highly Healthy Person
Copyright © 2003 by Walt Larimore

Requests for information should be addressed to:
Zondervan, *Grand Rapids, Michigan 49530*

Library of Congress Cataloging-in-Publication Data

Larimore, Walter L.
     [10 essentials of highly healthy people]
     God's design for the highly healthy person / Walt Larimore, with Traci Mullins.
     "Formerly titled: 10 essentials of highly healthy people."
        p. cm.
     Includes bibliographical references and index.
     ISBN 0-310-26279-8 (softcover)
     1. Health.   2. Health — Religious aspects — Christianity.   3. Health behavior.
I. Mullins, Traci, 1960–   II. Title.
RA776.L3496 2004
613 — dc21

                                                2004019428

Interior design by Tracey Walker

Printed in the United States of America

---

04 05 06 07 08 09 10 /❖ DCI/ 10 9 8 7 6 5 4 3 2 1

To Maxine and Larry,
Pud and Stan—
with eternal thanks
for providing Barb and me
with a highly healthy family and home

Dear Reader,

We have needed this book for a long time. Bookstores are full of health care books, but this book isn't like them. And there are dozens of Internet Websites that propose to answer every conceivable question about your health. While these resources provide lots of information, few attempt to give the insight you need to become and stay highly healthy. As a physician who works with thousands of doctors across the country, I'm convinced that too few health care professionals know or apply the information found in Dr. Larimore's book.

While we are a more health-*conscious* society, we seem to be less healthy than our parents and grandparents. Yes, we have designer drugs for every health dilemma. Antibiotics can cure most of the infectious diseases that killed earlier generations. Our hospitals are full of the latest high-tech gizmos to diagnose and treat our ailments. Yet, the complexity of health care sometimes is more harmful than helpful. We may be living longer than previous generations, but we don't sense we are healthier or better cared for. Health is not just an absence of illness or an increased life span. As you will learn, it is much more than that.

Dr. Larimore shares the wisdom he has gleaned from decades of practice. You will learn practical tools to assess how spiritually, relationally, emotionally, and physically healthy you are. More important, you will learn proven and practical strategies to improve your health and relate to your doctor. If you apply what is taught here, it will transform your life.

The Christian Medical Association, with its 16,000 members, highly endorses this book. Our goal is to change the face of health care by changing the hearts of doctors. We are trying to create the kind of doctor you want— one who is competent and compassionate and who possesses the character of Christ. Dr. Larimore is just that kind of physician. He is a doctor's doctor— the kind of doctor other physicians want for their own family members. You couldn't have a better guide for learning the *essentials of healthy living*.

Ready to begin your journey? Find a comfortable chair—once you start reading, you won't want to stop. Grab a highlighter to mark the information you won't want to forget. And don't forget to write your name in the front. You are sure to loan it to a friend. Better yet, give it to him or her. It's one of the most important gifts you could give to someone you love.

—David Stevens, M.D., executive director
Christian Medical Association

Contents

Foreword

Dr. Walt Larimore is the same doctor of family medicine we doctors and medical students came to know and love a few years back when he produced a training course called "The Saline Solution." Walt took this seminar across America to teach doctors and medical students how to practice medicine in a "salty" way—referring to Jesus' command to be "the salt of the earth"—and to show how the practice of medicine could give doctors opportunities to minister to the mind and spirit, as well as to the bodies, of their patients.

Early in his career Walt practiced family medicine in a rural environment in a small town in the Smoky Mountains (read his *Bryson City Tales*). Later he moved to Kissimmee, Florida. During his more than twenty years of experience as a family physician, Walt became more and more impressed with the close relationship between the physical health of his patients and their mental, emotional, and spiritual background. He's come to realize that patients need to understand the essential *oneness* of their own minds and bodies.

So *this* book is for patients. Patients must learn to take the initiative and talk to their doctors about their fears and their relationships—and even about their faith. If their doctors turn out to be impatient—quick to prescribe treatment on the basis of primary physical symptoms alone—perhaps they're not the right doctor for them!

Walt Larimore wants you, the patient, to take charge of your own health. In the critical game of your life, learn to be your own quarterback! This book helps you understand yourself and teaches you to discover the disciplines that will make you highly healthy—including how to choose the right physician to work with you.

If you're afraid this will be heavy stuff, just begin reading. You'll find yourself laughing and crying over a whole fund of stories. You won't encounter highbrow medical terminology here; what you *will* find is a conversation with a trusted physician who realizes that most of his readers don't have medical training. In between his many stories you'll gain insights that reveal the great breadth and depth of Walt's experience and of his own reading, as he backs up his advice with reference to a wide range of excellent research.

Warning to doctors: Of course you wouldn't want to be seen reading a book for patients. However, I suggest you get a copy, smuggle it home, and read it in the closet. Otherwise you may find that your patients have the book and are ready to tell you things about how they can be highly healthy—things *you* should have been able to tell *them!*

—Paul Brand, M.D.

Acknowledgments

Many people have contributed to this book, but a few deserve special mention for their excellence and dedication. The staff at Zondervan has been wonderful. Cindy Lambert has become a confidante, cheerleader, encourager, equipper, and critic. Cindy's caring, her coaching and direction, and her friendship and hand-holding during every phase of the development of this book were critical. This book was inspired by her and named by her. Cindy is more than a superb editor; she has become a special friend.

Jane Haradine and Dirk Buursma pulled the final manuscript together. As a reader of this book, you will be the recipient of their commitment to high-quality editing and writing. Traci Mullins was more than a collaborating author for this work—she became a dear friend. Her frustrations at having to deal with a rookie author were legion. Yet her patience and kindness were never ending.

During my four years of practice in Bryson City, North Carolina, and my sixteen years in Kissimmee, Florida, my medical partners never ceased to teach me what it meant to be a physician who inculcates highly healthy habits into our patients. Rick Pyeritz, M.D., and John Hartman, M.D., were marvelous teachers, splendid partners, trusted confidants, and brilliant physicians. They were the family physicians for my family. Their love and care for the Larimores are forever appreciated and will never be forgotten. They are two of my dearest friends, and either could have written this book. Much of what you read here was cultivated while I was in practice with them.

During over twenty years of practice, I was privileged to care for thousands of patients. In many ways they were my most accomplished professors in what it means to be highly healthy. I have protected their privacy, even as I've shared some of their stories. I am so thankful to each of them.

A number of colleagues contributed to the concepts contained in this book. Thanks are due to David Aiken, M.D., Bruce Bagley, M.D., Dave Biebel, Scott Bolinder, Max Crocker, M.D., Tommy Dietz, Lloyd Duplantis, Michael Freeny, Len Fromer, M.D., Ken Grauer, M.D., Susie Hilsman, Sarah Jones, M.D., Gus Kinchen, Diane Komp, M.D., Dennis LaRavia, M.D., Joe Lieberman, M.D., M.P.H., Peter Nieman, M.D., Dean Patton, M.D., Robert Persons, M.D., Tim Trombitas, Mari Sanchez, M.D., Rafael Sanchez, M.D., Peter Saunders, M.D., Victor Sierpina, M.D., Curt Stine, M.D., Dick Tibbits, and Chip Watkins, M.D.

I owe a special debt of thanks to several colleagues whose teaching and wisdom are reflected in various sections of this book. My respect and admiration rest with Nikitas Zervanos, M.D., Harvey Elder, M.D., Don Hawkins, David Benware, Neil Brooks, M.D., Paul Williams, M.D., and Randy Alcorn.

My executive assistant, Donna Lewis, unselfishly assisted in manuscript review and research arrangements. Thanks, Donna. Thanks also to Mark Maddox and John Perrodin for reviewing the manuscript and making valuable suggestions.

I am so grateful to Randy Frazee for assisting me in adapting his Christian Life Profile to be used as a Spiritual Life Profile. Thanks, Randy. I owe George Barna a thank-you for allowing me to use his spiritual assessment tool. Thanks also to Dr. Redford Williams and Reid Boates for helping me obtain permission to use The Relationships Questionnaire.

I am indebted to the Christian Medical Association for their initiative in bringing this project to print. David Stevens, M.D., and Gene Rudd, M.D., through their leadership roles in this valuable organization, saw the need among Christian doctors and patients and were actively involved in bringing this project to fruition.

I am grateful to the Professional Review Committee organized by the Christian Medical Association—made up of primary care physicians in private practice and in academic medicine—that spent countless hours reviewing the manuscripts. Rick Kivosky, M.D. (Family Medicine, Indianapolis, Indiana), Grat Correll, M.D. (Family Medicine, Bristol, Tennessee), and Gene Rudd, M.D. (Obstetrics and Gynecology, Bristol, Tennessee) volunteered significant amounts of their time to go through this book in great detail, evaluating and critiquing its medical content. Their invaluable suggestions have improved this book immensely.

My deepest professional acknowledgment is due my good friend David Larson, M.D. Before his untimely death in 2001, David founded and led the National Institute of Healthcare Research. We met during my residency at Duke in the late 1970s and then lost contact until the early 1990s, when David became a mentor for my research, speaking, and writing on the topic of spiritual care in clinical medicine. He was generous with his time and teaching. His friendship was a priceless gift.

I also want to acknowledge the love, prayers, support, and encouragement of my best friend of over forty-five years and my wife of twenty-nine years, Barb. All she's done and sacrificed to make it possible for me to write cannot be overstated. Barb, I love you.

Finally, I am grateful to God for allowing me to serve him through writing. My deepest prayer is that this work will bring glory to him and his health to you.

Walt Larimore, M.D.
Colorado Springs, Colorado
October 2002

Meet Dr. Larimore

I never wanted to be a doctor. In fact, I never even thought about it—at least not until the idea was put into my head by someone I had known for many years. Dr. Stan Shaw was a lifelong educator, as was his wife, Inez (friends call her Pud). Stan and Pud both taught in Baton Rouge, Louisiana. They loved teaching, they loved children, and they had keen insight to recognize what made their students tick.

I had met Stan and Pud's oldest daughter, Barbara, when she and I were kindergartners. (By the way, this same Barb is my wife today. But I'm getting ahead of myself.)

During my first year of college, Stan saw within me something I had never seen—something I might have continued to ignore without his concern and encouragement. One day in his workshop, he posed a life-altering question: "Have you ever thought about going into law or medicine?"

I still remember feeling totally befuddled. I had never given these careers any serious thought. I had never seen myself as capable of doing either. "I think you'd be really good in either field," Stan said. "I think these professions really fit the type of person you are."

That was all he said. But it was enough to bring back some significant and precious memories. During my childhood, my mother had been a nurse in the labor and delivery unit at a local hospital. On weekends, she worked the 3:00 P.M. to 11:00 P.M. shift. By the time she got home, my younger brother, Billy, and I would usually be fast asleep. But many nights after work, she'd sit on my bed and tell me about her "deliveries." She'd recount both the blessings and the tragedies of that particular shift. She felt called to her vocation. She loved being a nurse, and she loved her patients. She admired many of the physicians with whom she worked. I'd hear stories about their compassion and the excellent care they provided—but I'd also hear about those who were . . . well, dare I say, less than "excellent."

Putting Mom's example and Stan's encouragement together was all the motivation I needed at that juncture in my life. The next semester I changed my major from marine biology to premed. And it was during my senior year that Stan and Pud allowed me the privilege of marrying their oldest daughter.

In August 1974, I entered medical school at Louisiana State University in New Orleans (I call it "Harvard on the Bayou"). Barb put me through school, working as a teacher. Medical school was followed by a teaching fellowship at the Queen's Medical Center in Nottingham, England, and then a time of traveling around continental Europe. After that, we settled into my residency in family medicine at Duke University Medical Center in Durham, North Carolina. All was well in our world—or so we thought.

A ROCKY ROAD TO WHOLENESS

It was in Durham, during my first year of residency at Duke, that the difficulties of life began to encroach. My left lung repeatedly collapsed, finally resulting in major surgery to remove part of my lung, followed by a stay in the intensive care unit. During my slow and painful recovery period, Barb was pregnant with our first child. When Kate was born, she had only 30 percent of a normal brain. Because of her severe cerebral palsy and a seizure disorder, we were given the devastating news that she would never walk or talk.

Raising a severely handicapped child put a tremendous burden on our lives, and our marriage suffered immeasurably. We made a very unwise investment resulting in a debt equal to over a year's salary, which took us nearly five years of labor and hardship to settle. Then Barb and I walked through the unthinkable horror of losing four children to miscarriage. Three of the miscarriages occurred in the middle of the pregnancy, after Barb had experienced the soaring hope of new life with each one, having felt each tiny person move and kick.

We were learning firsthand about suffering and sadness, disappointment and despair. Thoughts of divorce and near bankruptcy played with our minds. We prayed for our daughter's complete healing, but our prayers were answered with a soft but sure, "No."

Although parts of our life together were proving to be painful and perplexing, there was an anchor that secured us through it all. That anchor—our personal relationship with our Creator and our faith in his goodness—is deeper today than ever before, as it continues to offer comfort and hope in spite of our circumstances. Not only have we been able to cope with our burdens, but we believe we've become more mature and healthier than we ever could have become had life's path been smooth and easy. In fact, we're convinced we're healthier at fifty-something than at any previous point in our lives.

Carrying these life experiences into the medical examining room or the birthing suite or the operating room or the emergency room has resulted, I believe, in my becoming a different physician than I would have been without them. My training in medicine was superb. I was intellectually prepared by many fine teachers, professors, and mentors to be a competent physician. However, wrestling with life and with the Author of life is what forged me into a family physician who has had the privilege and joy of helping my patients become highly healthy—not just physically but emotionally, relationally, and spiritually as well.

During countless hours over two decades of practicing medicine, I've had the unrivaled gratification, as the attending physician during the birth of more than 1,500 children, to place these precious gifts into the arms of their moms. I've treated many patients through the rigors of both acute and chronic illness. I've set bones, stitched up lacerations, and operated on ruptured appendixes and sick gall bladders. On too many occasions I've had to tell a person he or she has cancer or an incurable disease. I've counseled couples as they've tried to pick up the pieces of shattered dreams. I've had to walk into emergency room lounges to tell a family that their child, their loved one, did not survive. I've had to pronounce patients dead, counsel with their families, and then attend their funerals. I've also had the high privilege of praying with many of these patients and families. I've seen many begin their own personal relationship with God. I've watched some learn what it means to be not just healthy but highly healthy. Not all have wanted to learn or been willing to invest the effort, but those who have accepted the challenge have been changed in profound ways.

All of these experiences have served to inform and mold my view of health and health care—of life and living. My research, teaching, and writing, my work in the media, and my travels have given me a unique view of highly healthy living—a view supported by medical evidence and the proven wisdom of the ancient Scriptures. This view recognizes that your body, your mind, your emotions, your spirit, your family and friends and faith community, your caregivers, and your Creator are all essential to your becoming as healthy as possible. I hope you will find this unique view of health helpful as you seek your own path toward becoming a highly healthy person.

First we'll chat about you for a while, as I help you evaluate your health—today. I'll review some stunning medical research. I'll look at the most significant of the ancient insights about health and healing. Page by page, I'll unpack the multifaceted answer to the basic question, "What is health?" You'll learn what you can do to be not only healthy (or healthier) but *highly healthy.* You'll learn what will make your journey through life not only better but also more satisfying—richer and more meaningful and worthwhile.

By the time you've considered the ten essentials of highly healthy people and begun to apply the "prescriptions" in these pages, you'll notice an important difference in your life. Your understanding of what *really* contributes to being highly healthy will change dramatically. You are about to discover that you have some surprising choices to make that will make you a highly healthy person.

Walt Larimore, M.D.
Colorado Springs, Colorado
October 2002

Getting the Most
Out of This Book

There are at least three ways to maximize the benefits of this book. The first option is to use this simple three-step approach if you need an immediate fix:

- ❖ Assess your health.
- ❖ Fix the spoke that's broke.
- ❖ Benefit from immediate action.

Simply complete the wheel assessment in chapter 2, which will help you find the spoke that's broke. Then, using the chart on page 39, read the section that's designed to help you fix the spoke that's broke. Finally, take the recommended action.

A second option is to read through the book to get an overview and then go back to the area of greatest need and drill down. A third option is to purchase a journal or notebook and carefully read and study the book, doing the assessments and considering applications as you go. No matter which option you choose, be prepared to spend time meditating, studying, learning, and praying.

USING A JOURNAL

Using a journal as you study this book can make the difference between good intentions and actually achieving the results you desire. By journaling you'll prioritize what you want to accomplish and make your goals as specific as possible.

Purchase a journal with blank pages. On the first page, write your name and the date you begin your journey toward nurturing your highly healthy teen. Keep the journal with your book, writing notes to yourself as you read. This journal is private—for your (and your spouse's) eyes only.

As you journal, note each principle and the action you're applying, as well as each goal you're setting. Give yourself plenty of time to accomplish each goal. Making progress toward your goals—even if it's steady and slow—is more important than setting goals you can't reach.

USING THE INTERNET RECOMMENDATIONS

At times I recommend information or resources that can be accessed easily via the Internet, but I haven't provided the Internet addresses for two reasons: (1) Web addresses tend to change over time, and (2) I may find better sites in the future. Therefore, I built an Internet site (www.highlyhealthy.net) you'll be able to visit at no cost. At www.highlyhealthy.net, you'll find a list of each of the sites I've recommended. By double-clicking on these listings, you'll be taken to the most up-to-date site for the information or health tools you need.

This site will be updated as often as needed and will host not only *God's Design for the Highly Healthy Person*, but also *God's Design for the Highly Healthy Child* and *God's Design for the Highly Healthy Teen*, as well as any other *Highly Healthy* tools, books, or newsletters that may be developed in the future.

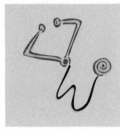

PART ONE

ASSESSING
YOUR HEALTH

CHAPTER ONE

What Is a Highly Healthy Person?

A s I hung up the phone, I groaned.

"Dr. Larimore," she had said sweetly, "this is Miss Bingingham. I teach the second grade at Bryson City Elementary School over here on School House Hill."

(I was learning that every hill in Bryson City, North Carolina, was named in this manner. My office was at the foot of Hospital Hill. Guess what was on top of that one?)

It was November 1981. My wife, Barb (seven months pregnant), and I, along with our three-year-old daughter, Kate, had just moved to this tiny town of about a thousand souls at the southern entrance to Great Smoky Mountains National Park to begin my chosen profession as a family physician.

Miss Bingingham said, "Every Thursday we try to have someone give a brief talk to our class. Would you be able to come and talk to the students about health? You know, tell the kids what health is and what they can do to keep their health."

She caught me off guard. I immediately thought of a thousand excuses. However, before I could verbalize even one, she said, almost in a whisper, "Doc [the folks in Bryson City liked to call health care professionals "Doc"—even the senior pharmacist at Swain County Drug Store was "Doc John"], some of the kids I teach aren't the brightest. But I think they'd really like to meet you, and I know they could learn a lot from you. Will you consider coming?"

I was sunk. What excuse could be good enough?

"Yes," I gulped. "I'd be delighted."

My mind started reeling. How could I explain to a bunch of second graders what health is when I wasn't sure what it was in my own mind? During medical school, I had been taught to recognize and treat diseases. I had had very little training in keeping people healthy and even less on how to motivate people to become healthy.

I've never forgotten that day, although I don't have a clue what I said in my little talk. I do remember that the kids listened politely. They even clapped. They asked lots of questions. I think I knew the answers. But even now, more than twenty years later, I wonder what they heard. Are they healthier because of their brief interaction with me? I doubt it. But I am. On that day I began to think more about ways I could promote health, not just treat sickness. I realized I needed to learn more, so I could help people gain health and satisfaction in their lives.

HEALTH AND WHOLENESS

Many people who came to me for medical care were highly unhealthy. One of my favorite examples of "unhealthy" comes from the movie *City Slickers,* in the scene where Mitch Robbins (played by Billy Crystal) is asked to make a presentation to his son's class about his occupation. Instead, he gives a brief oration that describes his view of life (and of his health):

> Value this time in your life, kids, because this is the time in your life when you still have your choices, and it goes by so quickly. When you're a teenager, you think you can do anything, and you do. Your twenties are a blur. Thirties? You raise your family, you make a little money, and you think to yourself, *"What happened to my twenties?"* Forties? You grow a little potbelly, you grow another chin, the music starts to get too loud, one of your old girlfriends from high school becomes a grandmother. Fifties? You have a minor surgery. You'll call it a procedure, but it's a surgery. Sixties? You'll have a major surgery, the music is still loud, but it doesn't matter because you can't hear it anyway. Seventies? You and the wife retire to Fort Lauderdale, start eating dinner at two o'clock in the afternoon, you have lunch around ten, breakfast the night before. You spend most of your time wandering around malls looking for the ultimate soft yogurt and muttering, "How come the kids don't call? How come the kids don't call?" The eighties? You'll have a major stroke. You end up babbling to some Jamaican nurse who your wife can't stand but who you call mama. Any questions?

Can you imagine such a cynical view of life—of health? Yet over the last two decades I've encountered many patients who seem to think pretty much this way. By contrast, the patients who have expanded my understanding of health are those who are vivacious and full of life—and who *want* to become or stay highly healthy. They seem to live their lives with purpose, drive, and meaning, regardless of their circumstances.

One such patient was Terrie, an elementary school librarian. I was her physician for almost sixteen years—from her midlife, through menopause, and on into retirement. During that time she developed symptoms of diabetes and heart disease. Crippling arthritis slowed her down. Yet she always seemed to be on top of her game. She had a joie de vivre—an enjoyment of life. If you were to focus only on her list of physical problems, you'd say she had lost her health. Yet I came to realize that Terrie was one of my healthiest patients. Although her body was not operating as efficiently as it had earlier in her life, she learned how to manage her diseases and even improve her overall health. She was one of my first teachers of what it means to be highly healthy—not just disease- and symptom-free but *whole* in the most important ways.

Is physical health all there is to health? If you're in great physical shape, does that make you highly healthy? I don't think so. By the time you finish this book, I'm convinced you won't think so either.

HOW DO YOU DEFINE *HEALTH?*

If you had been asked to speak to Miss Bingingham's class about health, what would you have said? How would you explain what *health* is? Are people healthy if they don't feel sick? How healthy are *you?*

Here is a note from the wife of a man who "felt fine" and seemed to be in great emotional, spiritual, and relational health. But after a checkup, he got some bad news from his doctor. This is what his wife wrote:

> *My husband has been feeling great for years—and hadn't seen a doctor for almost a decade. In my usual tactful way, I told him last summer, "Hon, someone will have to sign your death certificate someday, and we need to get your name in someplace. You're coming up on seventy, so let's just both go and get physicals for 'baseline info.'"*
>
> *Turns out, while I'm fine, the doctor found that my husband has high blood pressure, high cholesterol, high glucose, and signs of possible colon problems. In mid-July he had to get two hearing aids. In mid-August he was operated on for Stage III colon cancer and is facing chemotherapy later. And just ten days ago (after further tests), he learned he has Type II diabetes and had to go on an oral diabetes medication. He's also on cholesterol and high blood pressure medications! Poor guy—he feels like he's*

*falling apart, even though he still feels okay physically (to our amaze-
ment). Emotionally we've both been through the wringer!*

Three months later, this man was dead—from diseases that could have been prevented or controlled if only he had committed at an earlier age to become highly healthy.

Or consider Cameron. Cameron focused on physical health. In fact he recently completed the Ironman triathlon, an amazing physical accomplishment. He is in top physical condition, physically disease-free yet struggling with severe depression. He focused so completely on physical fitness that essentially he had no friends and no social life. His wife and kids left him, and his business collapsed. Was it healthy for him to be at his physical prime yet unable to care about much of anything emotionally?

For a time, I provided medical care for prisoners in the county jail. Many had bodies that were healthy, yet a few described the sick pleasure they had experienced while raping or robbing or murdering someone. Some were totally unrepentant, and I was convinced that if they ever got out, they'd commit another crime. They had disease-free bodies, but were they highly healthy?

My training in conventional medicine initially led me to emphasize the physical side of health, particularly the treatment of trauma and illness. I viewed patients as healthy if they were free from diseases and injuries. But the more experience I gained, the more I could see that having a physically functioning body is not all-important. It isn't even the main factor in being a highly healthy individual. What, then, is the connection between physical well-being and total health?

WHOM SHOULD YOU TRUST TO DEFINE *HEALTH?*

What motivated you to pick up this book? What results are you hoping for? Obviously, you want to be highly healthy. Before you can take some steps to achieve this goal, you need to be sure you've *defined* the goal. Whom do you trust to define *health?*

Let's take a look at three sources and compare their opinions: first, the conclusions of current health care providers around the world; second, a few definitions from throughout history; and third, the definition provided by the World Health Organization, a group that has influenced health care around the world since 1948.

Current Health Care Providers

In preparing to write this book, I informally surveyed more than a thousand physicians and health care experts in many different countries. I asked them two questions: "What is health?" and "What are the essentials of health?"

After cataloging their surprising responses, I began to search the medical literature from around the world. I reviewed scores of studies and medical reports (many of which I'll refer to in the upcoming pages). I especially examined studies that focused on wellness and longevity. I looked at the histories of men and women who had lived a long time or who lived well to discover what kept them in this state of being highly healthy. Their stories and the data I cataloged all revolved around the same themes. All the evidence suggests that living well and living a long time involve a powerful connection between our physical bodies and our emotional, mental, relational, and spiritual well-being.

Historic Definitions of Health

In medical libraries there is a great deal of information on how ancient physicians, philosophers, and clergy defined health. I've noticed certain trends in writings that go back many centuries.

Our word *health* is said to be derived from an old English word that means "whole." The definition of health is intended to include those things that "make a person whole." Obviously, this means much more than just physical well-being.

Some ancient writers taught that hard work—both physical and mental—would result in health. One school of thought emphasized that work is compatible with improving health as long as it is *ego-syntonic*. In other words, work must be coupled with "enthusiasm" to be healthy. By implication, work that could not be done enthusiastically—work that was depressing, in other words—would actually steal from one's health.

Eighteenth-century authors posited the view that a calm temperament or tranquil spirit was a key to true health. Many associated health with a good sense of humor and an ability to laugh at oneself.

In their attempt to define health, some philosophers and physicians pointed to the Greek word *praus* ("gentle, meek")—a quality they promoted as a virtue of high order. According to Aristotle, *praus* had to do with one's ability to temper the feeling of anger, or what he called *thymos*. The ancient Greeks used the term *thymos* to describe a force that boiled or welled up or "went up in smoke." Therefore, to the Greeks this quality called *praus* was one's ability to acquire an even temperament. *Praus*, the Greeks claimed, created much good health and very little ill effect on others or on oneself.

Many modern-day writers and physicians have wrestled with the meaning of health and how to achieve it. Like the ancients, virtually none equate health with physical health alone. Historically it has meant much more.

The World Health Organization's Definition of Health

In 1948 a modern definition of health was included in the constitution of the fledgling World Health Organization (WHO):

> Health is a state of complete physical, mental, and social well-being and not merely the absence of disease or infirmity. The enjoyment of the highest attainable standard of health is one of the fundamental rights of every human being without distinction of race, religion, political belief, economic, or social condition.

In 1984, the WHO added *spirituality* to its list of factors necessary for optimum health.

The WHO definition was, at least in part, created as a reaction against certain modern definitions of health that neglected the emotional, social, and spiritual factors associated with human well-being. I considered the WHO definition of health as being on target—but in my heart of hearts I wasn't sure the definition was adequate.

A doctor who practices in an inner-city neighborhood articulates my perspective when she says, "[Unlike the WHO definition of health,] I think that true health involves our entire beings. The physical, mental, and spiritual elements must all be functioning as God designed them to function if we are to be truly healthy. The physical may actually be the most unimportant of the three, because with good mental and spiritual health we can still be content, even though our bodies may be unhealthy."

As you can see, multiple "authoritative" sources from ancient to modern times indicate that health is continually defined in terms of physical, emotional, mental, relational, and spiritual well-being.

Spiritual? you ask. *Are you saying I can't just focus on physical health? Why isn't that enough?* You will discover in these pages that our spirituality is key to becoming highly healthy persons and has a profound effect on our physical health.

So I have a rather bold suggestion to make. I'm going to recommend that, in addition to paying attention to thousands of medical studies, current medical advice, and historical medical wisdom, we also consider a book with proven timeless principles that can be applied in any culture at any time, a book that can teach patients the essentials they need to know in order to become highly healthy. Millions around the world refer to it as "The Good Book." That book is the Bible.

You've got to be kidding! you may be thinking. *How can a book that is thousands of years old be of any use in our era of science and modern medicine?*

To be highly healthy you have to think way beyond your body. Looking at what "The Good Book" has to say about health can give us some clues as to what makes up a high degree of overall health.

I admit I'm not a trained theologian. But as a student of the Bible for more than thirty years, I am familiar with many of its precepts and principles. I have become convinced that this ancient book of wisdom contains timeless principles of health that are *supported by scientific research.* Let's take a look.

WHAT THE BIBLE SAYS ABOUT HEALTH AND HEALING

In the Bible, health is viewed as completeness and wholeness. In his book *The Bible and Healing,* John Wilkinson, a British physician who was both a medical missionary and a biblical scholar, says that while the Bible appears to say little about health as defined in strictly medical or mental terms, "human wholeness or health is the main topic of the Bible. . . . It is only when human beings are whole and their relationships right, that they can be described as truly healthy."

Health in the Bible is a multifaceted concept. The Hebrew word *shalom,* while sometimes connoting "peace," is not just the absence of conflict, just as health is not just the absence of disease. Its root meaning is that of wholeness, completeness, and general well-being—but not just physical, emotional, and spiritual well-being. It also carries a strong emphasis on relational well-being, especially with regard to one's relationship with God. In fact, the Bible teaches that true *shalom* comes only from God: "The LORD gives strength to his people; the LORD blesses his people with peace." The Bible seems to indicate that one cannot be highly healthy physically, emotionally, and relationally unless one is also growing spiritually.

Also in the ancient Hebrew Scriptures is the root word *rapha,* which more than any other word describes the process of healing. The various noun and verb derivatives of this root occur at least eighty-six times in the Bible's Old Testament. The variety of uses of *rapha* tell us that God's activity as healer is not limited to the physical realm. He is depicted as wanting to restore every aspect of a person's life—physical, mental, social, and spiritual.

The Bible uses various terms to describe health broadly and comprehensively. King Solomon connects emotions to physical health: "A cheerful heart is good medicine, but a crushed spirit dries up the bones." King David poignantly describes how guilt over wrongdoing affects physical, spiritual, and emotional health. After committing adultery and murder, David wrote,

"When I kept silent, my bones wasted away through my groaning all day long. For day and night your hand was heavy upon me; my strength was sapped as in the heat of summer." The apostle John links our overall well-being to our spiritual vitality: "Dear friend, I pray that you may enjoy good health and that all may go well with you, even as your soul is getting along well."

Health is a major topic in the Bible, and it is viewed primarily as the restoration and strengthening of one's personal relationship with God. It is also viewed as a healthy lifestyle (physically and emotionally) that focuses on pursuing healthy relationships with your family and with other people.

A TIMELESS PERSPECTIVE ON TRUE HEALTH

The biblical view on health can be summed up with the word *blessed.* Blessedness is a theme in the Old Testament and is most clearly described in the New Testament in Jesus' Sermon on the Mount. The Bible makes the bold assertion that people who aren't socially, financially, physically, or mentally gifted can be blessed by God, not rejected by him, and as a result their overall health is enhanced.

Our overall health depends not just on our physical health, important as that is, but also on our inner life. It is this inner emotional and spiritual life that God most wants to nourish and promote, for he knows that without spiritual and emotional well-being, we are less healthy than we were designed to be.

Why am I stressing this timeless biblical view? Does it really matter in the twenty-first century? I believe it does. I've had many patients who were physically healthy, yet were social, emotional, and spiritual disasters, unable to grasp what it means to be highly healthy. I've had patients who have suffered trauma and disease, leading to chronic disability or pain or fatigue, who suffer daily—in ways most of us could not begin to imagine—yet who have been able to develop strategies for becoming highly healthy. I've also had patients (and a daughter) who live with permanent disability from a birth defect or congenital disease, whose prayers for healing have been answered in ways they never would have imagined.

From all this I have come to believe that being healthy—truly healthy—is *not* dependent on physical well-being alone. Being highly healthy means being healthy in every area of your life during every stage of your life. It means being balanced in these areas: body, mind, spirit, and community—what I call the four "wheels" of health—which you will be putting to the test in the next chapter. By balancing these aspects of health, you can become blessed and, thus, highly healthy.

LET'S GET PRACTICAL

Are you ready for a few surprises? Within these pages you'll find a number of practical and reasonable choices you can make that can improve your health.

This book draws on the latest medical research, as well as on stories and experiences of physicians and patients from around the world. And it unashamedly uses the health-related principles from "The Good Book" as one of its foundations. Through these sources and my experience in medical practice, I've found ten principles that I believe are essential to being highly healthy. At first glance you may suspect that these essentials don't have much impact on your physical health. You're about to discover otherwise.

1. The essential of balance
2. The essential of self-care
3. The essential of forgiveness
4. The essential of reducing SADness (stress, anxiety, and depression)
5. The essential of relationships
6. The essential of spiritual well-being
7. The essential of a positive self-image
8. The essential of discovering your destiny
9. The essential of personal responsibility and empowerment
10. The essential of teamwork

These essentials are designed and programmed into the very core of our beings. If you understand them and learn to apply them in your life, you will be taking the first steps to becoming highly healthy. Putting into practice the essentials explained in the rest of this book is . . . well . . . essential.

CHAPTER TWO

Testing Your Four Wheels of Health

L eona was dying of cancer. I had treated more than a few terminally ill patients over the years, but Leona stood out. She faced death head-on—courageously and even joyfully. Her family drew strength from her as she died. In over two decades of practicing medicine, she was one of my most highly healthy patients.

On the other hand, one of the unhealthiest patients I ever treated was a great athlete whose family life was in shambles and his business a wreck.

If you ask most folks to tell you which of these two was healthiest, their answer would be wrong.

Many of the physician-respondents to my informal survey commented on patients who suffered from poor physical or mental health, yet were highly healthy people. One doctor told me about a patient who, in the prime of his adult life, became paralyzed from the neck down in an accident, yet who exudes hope and enthusiasm and maintains rich family and social relationships. "The essence of true health," this doctor wrote, "is physical, emotional, social, and spiritual well-being. When these four dimensions are singing in harmony, you're healthy. That doesn't mean there's no room for a dissonant chord, but that the music of life is pleasant to the ear. My quadriplegic patient seems to me to be highly healthy, despite his sobering physical disability."

I, too, have spoken with many seriously disabled or diseased people who seem healthier than I am. What they all share is a conscious and continuous effort to seek the highest possible degree of health in four distinct aspects of their lives.

Which brings me to Harold. Funny, I hadn't thought about him for more than twenty years. But as I was considering my definition of being highly healthy, Harold came to mind. Through the mountains near Bryson City, North Carolina, runs the Nantahala River. A number of somewhat eccentric folks live in the hollows above the hordes of tourists who raft down the white water. Harold was one of these modern-day mountain men. He lived alone in a small cabin on a hill above the river.

Harold had been a lawyer, but he became disillusioned with the practice of law and set up his new life in the mountains. He made his money serving as a river guide with one of the local rafting companies. But his true joy was in refurbishing old Model T Fords. He labored over repairing their bodies and reupholstering their seats. But his specialty was repairing their wheels. They didn't look like much to me, but to Harold they were works of art.

One day Harold invited me to his shop, where he waxed eloquent about wheels. He showed me how a weakness in just one or two of the spokes could cause the wheel to collapse—and potentially cause a wreck. He explained how the wheels had to be as perfectly balanced as possible—at least if the driver wanted a long, smooth ride. He demonstrated how even one wheel out of alignment can put a strain on the engine, the chassis, and the other wheels. In short, an imbalance in one wheel can goof up the whole car.

I began to think of the components of health in the way Harold taught me to think of the components of a sturdy wheel: four wheels to a stable car (four health "wheels" of a highly healthy person), strong spokes for each wheel, all wheels in balance.

Interestingly, four components run through the definitions of health given by many ancients and by the contemporary experts with whom I consulted. They're also present in the latest scientific research and in the Bible. I believe the four health "wheels" of highly healthy people are

- **physical health**—the well-being of one's body;
- **emotional health**—the well-being of one's mental faculties and one's connection with his or her various emotions;
- **relational health**—the well-being of one's associations with family, colleagues, and friends in the context of a community that is healthy; and
- **spiritual health**—the well-being of one's relationship with God.

THE PHYSICAL WHEEL

What is physical health? To put it simply, maximum physical health happens when the body—with all its chemicals, parts, and systems—is functioning as closely as possible to the way God designed it to function. For a person to be physically healthy, disease must be prevented whenever possible and treated as needed. When illness or disorder is incurable, physical health involves learning to cope with and adapt to physical disease. Can you see, then, why the physical wheel may actually be the least important of the four? With good emotional, relational, and spiritual health a person can still be highly healthy, even though his or her body may not be "whole."

Our daughter, Kate, was born with cerebral palsy. A significant portion of her brain had died and dissolved while she was in the womb, leaving the left side of her body weakened and spastic. The brain damage slowed her physical development and required her to have many operations to straighten her limbs and her eyes. Although Kate, now twenty-five, is not "normal" physically, and her condition is incurable, she has learned to cope and adapt physically. I consider her physical wheel to be healthy—to be well-balanced. Even so, Kate's physical health is strongly dependent on her constant work to keep her emotional, relational, and spiritual wheels in balance.

THE EMOTIONAL WHEEL

Emotional health is the state of maximum emotional and mental wellbeing. I don't define this, however, as merely the absence of emotional distress—unavoidable for any imperfect human being. (That's all of us!) Being emotionally healthy requires learning to cope with and to embrace the full spectrum of human emotions each of us faces every day throughout our lives.

My friend Suzanne models what being highly healthy emotionally looks like. For many years I've watched her handle whatever life hands her. Now in her fifties, Suzanne is one of the most authentic people I've ever known. Whether she is experiencing the sudden jolt of loss, the sweet joy of dreams realized, or the ordinary ups and downs of daily life, she wholeheartedly *feels* the varied emotions associated with each. She doesn't pretend things are better than they are, nor does she consider the inevitable letdowns of human existence "catastrophes." She has a healthy relationship with her own emotional life, neither running from nor chasing down the lows and highs along her journey. Her willingness to lean into and experience the rich scope of human emotion inspires me to do the same, even when it's uncomfortable!

Being mentally healthy requires healthy brain function. Charles, a former patient, lives with a severe, inherited form of chemical depression. This brain dysfunction, when untreated, leaves him nonfunctional—it throws his physical, emotional, relational, and spiritual wheels out of balance. When he's at his worst, he loses his appetite, motivation, and concentration. But by taking a prescribed antidepressant medication, taking care of himself physically by eating right and by exercising, and proactively balancing his physical, relational, and spiritual wheels, Charles can reverse this chemical dysfunction that otherwise profoundly impairs his mental health.

THE RELATIONAL WHEEL

Relational or social health is the state of maximum well-being in all of our relationships—including those with family, friends, neighbors, coworkers, and our broader community. Does this mean living without any conflict? No. Relational stress and discord are inevitable as we interact with fellow human beings. It is critical to our overall well-being, however, to do all we can to prevent and "treat" disordered relationships.

Judy's spiritual wheel seemed intact, but she was a physical and emotional mess. As her doctor, I spent months trying to balance her physical and emotional wheels. No matter what I did for her medically (I tried every conceivable combination of treatments), she always came to my office out of balance.

I finally realized that her root disease stemmed not from physical or emotional disease but from a severely disordered and dysfunctional series of relationships. Only after she agreed to work on mending her relationships, with the help of a psychologist and a support group, could the other parts of her life become balanced. As Judy's relational wheel came into balance, she began to experience a smoother "ride," both physically and emotionally.

THE SPIRITUAL WHEEL

I define spiritual health as the state of maximum well-being in our personal relationship with our Creator. To be spiritually healthy, any separation or disharmony in our relationship with God must be prevented or treated. The spiritual wheel is in many ways the most crucial one, as good physical, emotional, and relational health will not by themselves allow us to become highly healthy people. Highly healthy people make their spiritual well-being a consistent priority. What does this mean? That they actively seek to understand God's plan and design for them in terms of their physical, emotional, relational, and spiritual condition. They seek and accept their Creator's personal instruction and direction in their lives.

Does this mean that physical, emotional, and relational health aren't important? Of course not. They can and should be enjoyed and appreciated. But keep in mind, if we give the spiritual wheel less attention than the other three, we cannot be highly healthy.

So what does it look like to have a healthy spiritual wheel? Consider the story of Margie. For a long time she was, in a word, neurotic! Not only that, she was in my office almost weekly. Her list of complaints, both imaginary and real, was long. These types of patients can be trying for any physician— simply because the patient chooses, either consciously or unconsciously, to never get well. They seem to know it, and the physician knows it.

I had taken a spiritual inventory during one of Margie's first visits to the office. I used what I call my **G-O-D** questionnaire, made up of three simple questions that allow me to get a sense of whether a personal relationship with God and a faith community is of importance to the patient.

I asked Margie the first question, the **G** question: "Is **G**od, spirituality, or religion of any importance to you, Margie?"

"Nope," was her curt reply.

I pressed on with the **O** question: "Do you ever meet with **O**thers in a faith community? Do you ever attend church or synagogue?"

"Nooooooo way!" was the shrill retort.

Honestly, I was fearful to ask the **D** question, but for the sake of completeness I pressed on, almost whispering: "Margie, is there anything I can **D**o to help you in your faith journey?"

"Are you nuts!?!" was all she could stammer between tightly pursed lips. I knew where she stood.

Despite the difficulty of caring for Margie, I found myself praying for her. And during office visits, I would occasionally suggest things I believed could change the course of her health. For example, one day I told her, "I know you don't think much about prayer, but I really believe it's effective. I've been praying that we'd find some treatment that would help you feel better."

She responded with a "Harrumph!"

One morning, when I walked into the exam room, she exploded from the chair with a hearty laugh and gave me a hug. (She had never done *that* before!)

"Margie, what are you so happy about? You seem almost giddy."

"Doc, you'll never believe it, but your prayers have been answered!"

"What are you talking about?" I asked.

She almost danced back to her chair. "I've begun going to church. Not 'cause I wanted to, mind you, but because my neighbor wouldn't stop inviting me! I went just to be neighborly. Well, you know what? I've learned some things about myself. I'm not saying I ever liked the way I was, but I never knew any other way. I tell you what, I don't know what happened, but something did, and I'm not the same woman!"

She looked me straight in the eyes. "Doc, thanks for praying for me and caring for me—but most of all, thanks for caring *about* me."

I didn't see Margie very often after that. My professional life was a bit easier, but a lot less salty!

Margie's case was fairly spectacular. Some might say she was healed. Indeed, I think she was—if not completely healed physically, at least transformed spiritually, relationally, and emotionally. Margie's experience demonstrates that all four wheels are connected. Admittedly, her case is only anecdotal (not the result of scientific research), but it illustrates the scientific evidence I'll share throughout the rest of the book. Like Margie, if you want to be highly healthy, you'll have to pay attention, making sure all four of your health wheels are inflated to the right pressure and well-balanced.

However, while balance in all four health wheels seems to be essential for achieving and maintaining the state of being highly healthy, the most important health wheel is the spiritual one. Can you see the value of learning to view your physical, emotional, and relational health as secondary to your spiritual health? While we're not promised a perfectly healthy physical life, the Bible promises those who have a vital relationship with God an abundant life, one that will be full and meaningful—infused with purpose, contentment, and joy. Because many groundbreaking studies show that spiritual health is so crucial, I'll talk more about it throughout the book—particularly in chapter 8.

ADJUSTING YOUR TIRE PRESSURE

"Walt," Barb inquired, "did you notice the nail in the tire of the car?"

I had not. So I took a look. All I could see was the head of the nail. It looked firmly embedded in the tire. No air was escaping—and we didn't have time to go get it fixed.

"Honey, I think we can keep going." Barb looked skeptical but nodded. About twenty miles later, the tire blew. Worse yet, the spare was flat! How I wished I'd heeded the warning and done what it would have taken to prevent a flat tire. My decision was neither wise nor practical.

Your four health wheels have many miles to travel. I want to focus on the *promotion* of health and the *prevention* of disease in each of your four health wheels. But simply scanning these pages won't produce results. To become a highly healthy person, you'll need to understand the four wheels of health and then take personal responsibility for your health.

I must warn you. You'll be tempted not to do what is needed to become highly healthy. It's very hard work. It takes time. You may be enticed by some health care providers who promise that their particular therapy will simply, easily, and quickly cure all that ails you.

Be on guard. It makes no more sense that any single "therapy" will restore your health than it does to think that a single mechanical intervention will keep your car running smoothly. Think about how complex cars are. They require regular checkups and preventive maintenance in order to avert problems. When they malfunction, they often require a professional's care—from a specialist who replaces mufflers to an expert to fix the transmission. The human body is hundreds of times more complex than any mechanical vehicle, and it requires even more care and special treatment.

Ready? Let's check you out.

HOW SMOOTH IS YOUR RIDE?

Each of the four health wheels has a hub and spokes. The hub—central to the entire wheel and the point around which the wheel turns—involves trust, or faith. I'm not speaking only in religious terms here but of the faith, confidence, assurance, and reliance you have that if you give your body what it needs to be healthy, it will respond by becoming healthier over time.

Each health wheel has at least two sets of spokes—the vertical and the horizontal—that are essential to a smooth ride. Understanding these wheels is fairly simple, and using them to evaluate yourself is pretty intuitive. The following exercise will help you quickly begin to get a handle on your health balance. On a separate sheet of paper reproduce or copy this simple illustration:

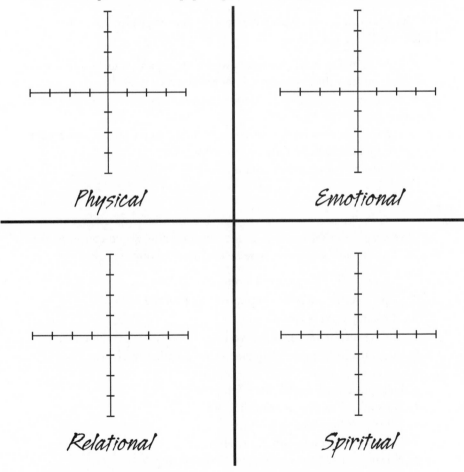

Physical

Emotional

Relational

Spiritual

You can download a complimentary copy of this illustration on the Web at www.highlyhealthy.net.

As you read each description below, make a mark on each spoke to represent your own evaluation of your individual spokes. As with each personal evaluation tool in this book, this evaluation is for *your* eyes only. The more honest you are with yourself, the more accurate these tools will be.

Physical Wheel

Hub = understanding one's body
Vertical Spokes = exercise and rest
Horizontal Spokes = nutrition/BMI and substance abuse/safety

Exercise

The top spoke on this wheel represents your average physical activity over the last two or three months.

- Full spoke: I exercise (run, walk, work out, or participate in sports activities) at least thirty minutes six or seven days a week.
- 3/4 spoke: I exercise at least thirty minutes per day, four or five days a week.
- 1/2 spoke: I exercise at least thirty minutes per day, three days a week.
- 1/4 spoke: I exercise only two days a week.
- No spoke: I am a couch potato.

Rest

On average, over the last two to three months, how would you assess your sleep and rest habits? Consider these factors for the bottom spoke:

1. I go to bed at a reasonable hour.
2. I get a restful night of sleep most nights of the week.
3. I usually wake up refreshed.
4. I have one or two days per week for a hobby, rest, and recreation.
5. I enjoy one or more adequate, restful vacations each year.

- Full spoke: I achieve all five of the above.
- 3/4 spoke: I achieve four of the above.
- 1/2 spoke: I achieve three of the above.
- 1/4 spoke: I achieve two of the above.
- No spoke: I achieve zero or one of the above.

Now let's turn our attention from the vertical spokes of the physical health wheel to its horizontal spokes.

Diet and Nutrition/BMI

Use the left-hand spoke to evaluate your diet and nutrition habits. Three-quarters of this spoke is for your nutrition, and one quarter is for your BMI.

For the largest portion of this spoke, evaluate your diet and nutrition habits. Consider these factors:

1. I drink plenty of water daily.
2. I eat at least two to four servings of fruits and three to five servings of vegetables daily.
3. I eat at least two nutritious meals per day.
4. I have minimal intake of caffeine and soft drinks.
5. I have minimal intake of saturated fats and highly processed foods.
6. I have fewer than two or three fast-food meals a month.

- 3/4 spoke: I do all of the above.
- 1/2 spoke: I do four or five of the above.
- 1/4 spoke: I do two or three of above.
- No spoke: I do zero or one of the above.

Go to www.highlyhealthy.net for a chart to help determine your BMI:

- 1/4 spoke: My BMI is normal (20 to 24.9).
- No spoke: My BMI is overweight (25 to 26.9) or extremely overweight (27 to 29.9) or underweight (18.5 to 19.9).
- Subtract 1/4 spoke if your BMI indicates obesity (30 or above) or extreme underweight (less than 18.5).

Substance Abuse/Safety

Consider these factors for up to half of the right-hand spoke:

- 1/2 spoke: I am rarely exposed to secondhand smoke, don't use tobacco products or illicit drugs, drink no or small amounts of alcohol, and don't misuse prescription drugs.
- 1/4 spoke: I am often exposed to secondhand smoke or occasionally use tobacco products or illicit drugs, drink moderate amounts of alcohol, and don't misuse prescription drugs.
- No spoke: I use tobacco products daily or I use illicit drugs, and I often drink alcohol excessively or misuse prescription drugs.

For the remainder of this spoke, consider these factors:

1. I almost always drive at or under the speed limit.

   2.   I always buckle up when I drive.
   3.   I have smoke and carbon monoxide detectors in my home.
   4.   I see a primary care doctor for regular checkups.
   5.   I see a dentist for regular checkups.

- 1/2 spoke: I achieve four or five of the above.
- 1/4 spoke: I achieve two or three of the above
- No spoke: I achieve zero or one of the above.

Emotional Wheel

Hub = understanding one's mind and emotions
Vertical Spokes = media/learning and work
Horizontal Spokes = stress/depression and hostility

To evaluate your emotional and relational wheels, you'll need to use the questionnaire in appendix 1 (page 261).

Media/Learning

To measure the top spoke, add together your exposure to media and your enjoyment of learning. Research shows that exposure to too much media or to the wrong type results in lower levels of health. Media can assault your senses, negatively affect your emotions, and become detrimental to your physical health. Rate your exposure to media as follows:

- 1/2 spoke: My home is TV free or I watch one hour or less a day, and I use the Internet less than one hour a day at home for non-work activity. And I never watch or am involved in pornographic or violent media.
- 1/4 spoke: I routinely watch or participate in one to four hours a day of media (television, videos, video games, and Internet/computer non-work activity at home). Or I sometimes watch or am involved in pornographic or violent media.
- No spoke: I routinely watch or participate in four or more hours a day of media (television, videos, video games, and Internet/computer non-work activity at home). Or I often watch or am involved in pornographic or violent media.
- Subtract up to 1/4 spoke if you have a TV in your bedroom or often eat in front of the TV.

The second half of the spoke is your enjoyment of learning and mental activity. As physical exercise helps your body stay healthy, your brain benefits from mental activity. Continuing to educate yourself and staying mentally active are ways to protect yourself from dementia and Alzheimer's disease. Mental activity through regular times of reading, doing crossword puzzles, playing board or card games, participating in ongoing education (attending an adult education class at church, auditing a community college course, for example), and having a challenging job is linked with a sharper mind later in life. Researchers have shown that the brain, like a muscle, must be exercised to remain highly healthy. Those who take the time to teach others what they know not only seem to have better health—especially emotional and mental health—they're also more likely to keep learning new things themselves.

So how much enjoyment do you receive from mental activities?

- 1/2 spoke: I have a moderate to high level of enjoyment for mental activities and learning.
- 1/4 spoke: I receive little or occasional enjoyment from mental activities and learning.
- No spoke: I receive no enjoyment from mental activities and learning.
- Add up to 1/4 spoke if you teach or coach others.

Work

The bottom spoke allows you to measure both the satisfaction you get from work and the proper amount of work. However, if you spend too much time at work—even when it's work you love—it can result in reduced physical and mental health.

What if you're retired? Measure your spoke by the meaningful volunteer work you do or the social, religious, hobby, or sport activities you participate in. If you're a full-time homemaker, just consider the first three factors below and take full credit for factor four!

1. My job is a good match and allows me to use my gifts, talents, and passions.
2. My work brings me a great deal of satisfaction.
3. I have good relationships with those with whom I work.
4. I routinely work less than fifty hours a week.

- Full spoke: I achieve all four of the above.
- 3/4 spoke: I achieve three of the above.
- 1/2 spoke: I achieve two of the above.
- 1/4 spoke: I achieve one of the above.
- No spoke: I achieve none of the above.

Stress/Depression

"SADness" (**S**tress, **A**nxiety, and **D**epression) dramatically decreases your health. While stress, anxiety, and depression are often unrecognized by those who suffer from them, the good news is that they can be treated. Use your stress and depression scores from appendix 1 to mark the left-hand spoke:

- Full spoke: My depression score is 0 or 1 and your stress score is 0.
- 3/4 spoke: My depression score is 2 or less or your stress score is 1.
- 1/2 spoke: My depression score is 3 or less or your stress score is 2.
- 1/4 spoke: My depression score is 4 or less or your stress score is 3.
- No spoke: My depression score is 5 or higher.

Hostility

For the right-hand spoke you'll need to use your hostility scores from appendix 1—which is a measure of anger, aggression, and cynicism. As I'll discuss in chapter 5, hostility kills. It's a highly unhealthy characteristic that is detrimental to your physical, emotional, relational, and spiritual health. Yet, like stress, anxiety, and depression, it can be treated.

- Full spoke: My hostility score is between 0 and 2.
- 3/4 spoke: My hostility score is between 3 and 6.
- 1/2 spoke: My hostility score is between 7 and 11.
- 1/4 spoke: My hostility score is between 12 and 16.
- No spoke: My hostility score is greater than 16.

Relational Wheel

Hub = understanding people and relationships
Vertical Spokes = parents/children and spouse
Horizontal Spokes = extended family/friends and social support

Parents/Children

The relationship you have (or had) with your parents plays a critical role in understanding who you are and in determining your emotional health and your ability to have good relationships. Apply the factors below to foster parents, adoptive parents, or grandparents if they raised you.

Children bring two obvious health benefits to their parents: first, the gratification of undertaking a significant work—the responsibility of raising another human being—and second, the companionship and joy that young people can bring into one's life. Children bring lots of work, worry, sacrifice, and stress, but along with it comes a healthy sense of purpose, significance, and connectedness—a sense of satisfaction from doing something important, which can have a profound impact on parents (or grandparents). Those who have never had children can gain a health benefit as well. Your relationship with any children who *are* in your life can help you become a highly healthy person. These "surrogate children" may be on a sports team you coach or part of a church youth group you lead; they may be the scouts you serve or the children of relatives or friends you care about and mentor.

Consider these factors in marking the top spoke:

1. My parent(s) balanced love with discipline.
2. My parent(s) balanced freedom with limits.
3. My parent(s) balanced nurture with training.
4. My relationship with my parent(s) when I became an adult was healthy, enjoyable, and affectionate.
5. I have children (or work with or care for children), and my relationship with them is meaningful and satisfying.

- Full spoke: All five of these are true in my life.
- 3/4 spoke: Four of these are true in my life.
- 1/2 spoke: Three of these are true in my life.
- 1/4 spoke: Two of these are true in my life.
- No spoke: Zero or one of these is true in my life.

Spouse

If you are married, ask your spouse, "On a scale of 1 to 4 [4 = outstanding], where would you rate our marriage right now?" Surprised? Or do you agree? A healthy marriage is a surprisingly strong predictor of high degrees of health.

If you are unmarried, it takes more work to become highly healthy. However, there are a couple of exceptions to this rule: (1) those who believe they are called by God to the single life and (2) those who are single but have a very satisfying nonsexual friendship with at least two friends or family members with whom they interact just about every day.

- Full spoke: I am married (and my spouse and I believe our marriage rates a 4), or I feel called to the single life or have a deeply meaningful, sexually pure relationship with at least two others.
- 3/4 spoke: I am married (and my spouse and I believe our marriage rates a 3), or I feel I'm called to the single life or have a deeply meaningful, sexually pure relationship with one person, or I'm widowed, separated, or divorced and have a deeply meaningful, sexually pure relationship with at least two others.

- 1/2 spoke: I am married (and my spouse and I believe our marriage rates a 2), or I feel I'm called to the single life and have no deeply meaningful relationships, or I'm widowed, separated, or divorced and have a deeply meaningful, sexually pure relationship with one person.
- 1/4 spoke: I am married (and my spouse and I believe our marriage rates a 1), or I'm widowed, separated, or divorced and have no deeply meaningful relationships.
- No spoke: I am married (and my spouse and I believe our marriage rates a 0).
- Subtract up to 1/4 spoke if you live with (cohabit) with someone. Research shows that the health benefits of a good marriage are not found among those who decide to live together.
- Subtract up to 1/2 spoke if you are or have been sexually active with someone other than your spouse.

Extended Family/Friends

Our relatives—sisters and brothers, aunts and uncles, cousins—can have a decidedly positive impact on our mental, physical, and spiritual health. Similarly, healthy friendships (people who love and care for us and who assure us of unconditional support) seem to be associated with higher levels of health.

For part of this left-hand spoke, consider the following:

- 1/4 spoke: My present relationships with my siblings or other extended family members are good to excellent.
- No spoke: My present relationships with my siblings or other extended family are nonexistent to poor.

For the rest of the left-hand spoke, consider these factors (add the two meaures together to score this spoke):

- 3/4 spoke: I have two or more dear friends with whom I interact frequently and who provide me great support and friendship.
- 1/2 spoke: I have one dear friend with whom I interact frequently and who provides me great support and friendship, or I have two or more friends with whom I interact occasionally to frequently but who don't always provide me the support I need.
- 1/4 spoke: I have no close or dear friends. My relationships seem to be superficial, or I have a relationship that is violent or hostile.
- No spoke: I'm a loner with little support or intimacy in my relationships, or I have two or more relationships that are violent or hostile.

Social Support

Apart from our genetic makeup, one of the most powerful across-the-board factors in predicting premature death and disease is lack of healthy social support. Those who believe no one really cares for them, who don't feel close to anyone, or who feel they have no one in whom to confide or to help them out of a bind are three to five times as likely to suffer premature disease or death. For this right-hand spoke, use the social support score from appendix 1. It is a measure of your emotional support, belonging support, tangible support, and self-esteem (the degree to which your relationships boost self-worth):

- Full spoke: My social support score is between 37 and 40.
- 3/4 spoke: My social support score is between 34 and 36.
- 1/2 spoke: My social support score is between 31 and 33.
- 1/4 spoke: My social support score is between 28 and 30.
- No spoke: My social support score is less than 28.

Spiritual Wheel

Hub = knowing God
Vertical Spokes = prayer and meditation
Horizontal Spokes = fellowship in a faith community and faith sharing

Prayer

Prayer is, in its simplest form, conversation with God. It can occur anywhere and at any time. It doesn't require a particular position. It's just an intimate discussion with someone who loves you more than you could ever imagine. Consider your experience with prayer in rating the top spoke:

- Full spoke: I pray once or more per day.
- 3/4 spoke: I pray a few days a week.
- 1/2 spoke: I pray a few times a month.
- 1/4 spoke: I pray infrequently (a few times a year).
- No spoke: I'm not a praying person or would pray only in a crisis.

Meditation

Meditation is all about listening to God. I've come to combine prayer and Bible reading with meditation. I see Bible reading and study as my listening to God speak. As I read and then "hear" God's whisper in my spirit, I talk back to him in prayer. At times, he and I are quiet—I simply meditate on what he's said. Other times I'll record our give-and-take through journaling. Consider these factors in rating the bottom spoke:

1. I meditate or read the Bible on a daily basis.
2. I routinely have a quiet time of reflection.
3. I keep a journal to record my thoughts and meditations.
4. I consistently memorize portions of the Bible (storing it in my heart).
5. I study the Bible quite frequently or participate in a Bible study once or twice a year.

- Full spoke: I achieve all five of the above.
- 3/4 spoke: I achieve four of the above.
- 1/2 spoke: I achieve three of the above.
- 1/4 spoke: I achieve one or two of the above.
- No spoke: I achieve zero or one of the above.

Fellowship in a Faith Community

The counsel of those who know you can be valuable. Having a spiritual accountability partner and being part of a small group of supporters who share your faith perspective and who unconditionally love you are critical aspects of keeping your spiritual wheel balanced. A common mistake is trying to go it alone spiritually. God has created us to operate best in community with others. When we love and encourage each other, teach and guide each other, correct and admonish each other, we become more quickly the people God created us to become. In rating this spoke, consider the following factors:

1. I consider my spiritual community to be loving and supportive.
2. I am an active member of a church or organized faith community.
3. I am involved with a small group of fellow believers who hold me accountable and give me positive, meaningful feedback, teaching, and fellowship.
4. I receive personal direction from at least one spiritual mentor.

- Full spoke: All four of the above are true.
- 3/4 spoke: Three of the above are true.
- 1/2 spoke: Two of the above are true.
- 1/4 spoke: One of the above is true.
- No spoke: None of the above are true.

Faith Sharing

For people of faith, a critical factor in balancing their spiritual wheel is to form and build relationships outside of their faith community. It allows them to exercise and share their faith. In marking this spoke, consider these factors:

1. I am actively involved with people outside my faith community.

2. I am generous in volunteering my time, treasure, and talent in the community in which I live and work.

3. My faith overflows through my competence at my work. In other words, I always try to do excellent work that glorifies God.

4. My faith overflows through my character and compassion. In other words, my life usually manifests love, joy, peace, patience, kindness, goodness, gentleness, faithfulness, and self-control.

5. My faith overflows through my communication with others, and I am comfortable sharing the principles of my faith with those who ask for or may need my help.

6. I am comfortable sharing the basic doctrines of my faith with those who ask or want to know about them.

- Full spoke: All six of the above are true.
- 3/4 spoke: Five of the above are true.
- 1/2 spoke: Four of the above are true.
- 1/4 spoke: Two or three of the above are true.
- No spoke: Zero or one of the above are true.

DRAWING YOUR WHEELS

Now that you've estimated the length of each spoke on each of the four wheels, go ahead and draw your wheels. Connect the end of each spoke with the one before and after it. How do the four wheels look. Are they round, or do they have flat sections? Are all four the same size, or is one much smaller?Are they all fairly round and about the same size, but with short spokes? If so, they'll turn far faster than they should, and you'll be at much greater risk to burn out.

More likely, one or more (perhaps all) of your wheels are different sizes— and not at all round. Can you imagine how a vehicle would run if it had four wheels like this? Probably not very well—and certainly not nearly as long as it should. And it'd be pretty bumpy indeed.

This exercise is designed to give a visual representation of overall health, so you can begin the process of lengthening the various spokes and improving your well-being. You may not encounter big surprises; rather, you may simply recognize and label much of what you suspected was true about yourself. Or you may be confronted with some surprises—and even a shock or two.

The illustration on the next page shows the assessment of a friend who was surprised at the condition of his wheels. "Walt," he said, "I'd say, 'Let's roll,' but I won't. So let's go to work!"

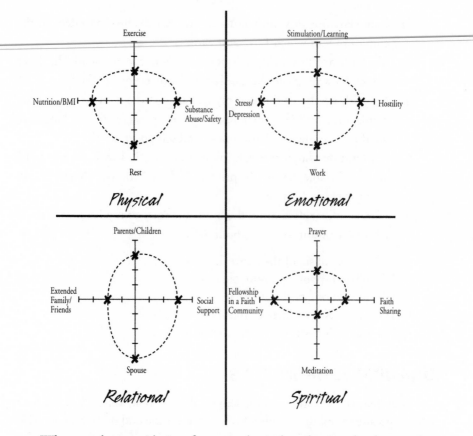

Whatever the case, it's time for you to begin lengthening the short spokes of your wheels. It's fine at this point to identify the flattest wheel or the most broken spokes. To find the flattest wheel, assign a point count to each spoke of each wheel. A full spoke gets 4 points, a 3/4 spoke gets 3 points, and half spoke gets 2 points, a 1/4 spoke gets 1 point, and no spoke gets 0 points.

A perfectly round, fully inflated wheel will have 16 points (4 points for each spoke). In this illustration, the physical wheel has 11 points, the emotional wheel has 12 points, the relational wheel has 12 points, and the spiritual wheel has 8 points. My friend's spiritual wheel is the least healthy, and it should probably be the first one he would address.

Another option is to deal with the shortest spoke(s). In this illustration, the bottom spoke on the spiritual wheel is the shortest. If you have more than one equally short spoke, choose the one that's easiest to address and read the section in the book that deals with that wheel of health.

It's time to go to work on your health. From this point on, you'll learn about each of the ten essentials of a highly healthy person and how you can apply them in your daily life.

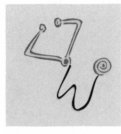

PART TWO

THE TEN
ESSENTIALS

CHAPTER THREE

Set a Wise Balance in Your Life

The Essential of Balance

I still remember my first car. Young men seem to have a propensity to remember their first vehicles—and I am no exception. That car was a two-tone 1958 Buick I bought for $100 after graduating from high school. It belonged to the grandparents of a close friend.

I remember caring for that car—washing it, changing the oil, keeping it clean and lubricated. And as is the case for anyone learning basic automobile care, I had to learn basic tire care. As long as the four tires were balanced and properly inflated, the car would roll along smoothly. But if one tire was unbalanced or improperly inflated, it would affect the entire vehicle. As my friend Harold taught me, this is especially true with regard to the simpler vehicles that have old-fashioned spoke wheels—like the Model T Ford. For a wheel to be healthy, it must have a healthy hub, a healthy set of spokes, and a healthy rim and tire.

Your "health car," with its four "wheels of health," simply cannot run smoothly without all wheels running well—being *in balance*. A car with unbalanced wheels might be able to run slowly and on smooth roads, but when the speed increases and the road gets bumpy, an unbalanced wheel can cause the car to swerve and career off the road. Neglecting one or more of your wheels of health will result in imbalance and health problems. It's like a wheel with uneven spokes—uneven and premature wear can and will take place.

If you discovered as you read the last chapter that your wheels are unbalanced (which they are sure to be unless you're some kind of superhero), then I welcome you to the human race! Don't beat yourself up or get discouraged. You simply can't attain balance in your life—you can't become a highly healthy person—without first *diagnosing* your unique areas of disease and imbalance. So hold your head up and focus your eyes straight ahead. There's encouragement and advice coming your way. The fact that you've gotten this far tells me that you truly want to be a highly healthy person—and that means there is great hope! As the old saying goes, "A journey of a thousand miles begins with a single step." You have begun the journey!

The following stories of people who have already fixed their health wheels (or are in the process of fixing them) will show you how it works.

PHYSICAL BALANCE

I first saw Hal for treatment of a chronic venous ulcer of the leg. Although he was only in his twenties, he had suffered with it for years—requiring several hospitalizations and surgeries. Hal was only five feet four inches tall, yet he weighed over 250 pounds. His nutritional habits were awful. He worked long hours in a sedentary job and suffered from a lot of on-the-job stress. He never exercised. The closest he ever got to physical activity was to click the TV remote control while watching others compete in football or basketball. He slept poorly—only a few hours a night—which left him feeling constantly tired and had a negative effect on his job performance.

Hal was chronically constipated and took in very little in the way of fluids, "except for a few Diet Pepsis while I'm working." He hated the way he looked and felt. Yet, apparently, he had never seen a physician who offered to help him become healthier.

My first order of business as Hal's doctor was to clear up the infection in the ulcer on his leg. However, I considered my job to have only begun. "Hal," I said, at the conclusion of what he thought would be his last visit to see me, "I know the ulcer has healed enough for you not to have to come back. But I'm concerned about your health. I think you are, too."

He nodded.

"Let's do something." I gave a brief and simple explanation of the physical wheel of health. I took out a piece of paper and drew a wheel with a hub, a wheel, and four spokes. Each spoke was marked with one-fourth, half, and three-fourths marks. I then handed him the paper and a pen. He went right to work. He and I already knew most of the answers, but drawing it out was a powerful illustration for both of us. He gave himself a half spoke for rest, a quarter spoke each for intake and elimination, and no spoke for activity.

Although I didn't completely agree with his assessment (I think I would have given him an eighth spoke for each of the four), it was important that Hal own this process and come up with his own assessment. If not, there'd be little chance he'd be motivated to make the necessary changes that could lengthen his spokes and improve his health.

"Based on this drawing," I said, "how does your physical health wheel look?"

He wouldn't look at me. He just stared at the drawing. Then he smiled and said, "Wow. It's flat." He paused for a moment. Then the smile left his face. He almost whispered, "It's real flat."

"Would you like to lengthen your spokes?"

Tears began to fill his eyes as he nodded.

"Let's make another appointment. When you come back, we'll go to work."

I gave him materials to study, and on the next visit he went to work on his physical wheel. What a joy it was for me, as his family physician, to see his wheel inflate over the years. The process was long and slow and tedious. But he did it. He *really* worked at it! Not only that, but over time we began working on his other three wheels as well.

Pick a Spoke—Any Spoke—and Lengthen It

Take a few minutes to note just *one* positive thing you can do to begin lengthening each of the spokes of your physical wheel. For example, will you take a day off this week and devote yourself to resting and rejuvenating? Will you drink eight glasses of water today? Start with *one* thing you can do to improve each spoke, and watch your wheel start to inflate!

EMOTIONAL BALANCE

I love to tell the story of Judith. Over the years she became not only a valued patient but also a precious friend. A successful businesswoman and fabulous mother of two beautiful daughters, Judith nevertheless was plagued by a large number of what we doctors call "nonspecific" complaints. She was fatigued, was sleeping poorly, and had decreased motivation at work. She was feeling more anxious and had recently experienced a couple of panic attacks. Her nine-year marriage was souring a bit, and her sexual appetite was waning.

Physically, other than being a tad overweight, she was in pretty good shape. Her physical wheel was nicely balanced. Mentally, her anxiety and familial dysthymia (chronic mild depression in Judith and several blood relatives) were fairly easily controlled with the appropriate medication. Yet, she told me, "I feel drained and unmotivated."

I still remember the day Judith and I sat down to talk about this—at a point when I was just beginning to understand the four wheels of health. As I explained the emotional parts of the wheel of health, I could see that the concept made sense to her. When I handed her the piece of paper with the wheel illustration, she went right to work. She gave herself a half spoke for stimulation, a fourth of a spoke for work, and no spoke for quiet or learning.

As she drew her spokes, she was smiling more and more. As she completed it and held it up for me to see, she exclaimed, "Bingo!" It was one of the most dramatic examples in my medical experience of what theologians call an epiphany. Judith instantly knew not only what the problem was but also what she needed to do about it.

Over the next few months, I saw her frequently for follow-up visits. Her slow but steady transformation was remarkable. After one of her appointments my nurse asked, "What are you prescribing for her?"

I smiled.

Judith used her flattened and unbalanced wheel as a starting point to steer herself toward a higher degree of health. She had several long talks with her husband, her priest, and her employer. She took another position at her workplace. Her salary went down a bit, but her satisfaction and job performance soared. As she learned new skills more closely aligned with her interests and temperament, she felt more intellectually stimulated and fulfilled.

Judith also started taking time to pamper and rejuvenate herself. She "scheduled" long, hot baths two or three times a week. She began to get up earlier to journal and enjoy some quiet time alone. On most days she'd take a short walk in the morning—"to exercise my body *and* my mind," she said.

About a year later, during her annual checkup, I had Judith draw her emotional wheel again. The spokes were not full-length, but getting close. Her wheel drawing reflected a better functioning and more functional woman— someone who was definitely becoming more highly healthy.

Judith isn't alone in feeling the stresses in the workplace. According to the Bureau of Labor Statistics, more than 25 million Americans work more than 49 hours each week. Of that number, 11 million spend 60 hours or more at work each week. Based on the sheer number of hours put in by Americans, one national newspaper gives the United States the dubious distinction of being "the most overworked nation in the industrialized world."

Researchers who study work environments blame long work hours for weakening ties with family and friends (the relational wheel) and also increasing the likelihood of work-related accidents (the physical wheel), as well as helping to bring about chronic stress, burnout, and anger or resentment (the emotional wheel). Even the American Medical Association now acknowledges that excessive work hours are not safe for young doctors or their patients. Some researchers warn that people who work long hours and then fail to get enough sleep once they get home could be putting their lives at risk. One study carried out in Australia and reported by the BBC suggested that the effects of sleep loss could be similar or even worse than the effects of drinking too much alcohol. Another study discovered that Japanese men who worked 61 hours a week or more on average during the previous year were twice as likely to have a heart attack as the men who worked 40 hours a week or less. They also found that the men who slept five hours or less on average each working day during the previous year had two to three times as great a risk of having a heart attack than men who got more than five hours of sleep.

Even death from working too many hours is being reported. In fact, *karoshi* is a Japanese word that means "death from overwork." The phenomenon was first identified in Japan, and the word is being adopted internationally. The evidence that overwork causes sudden death is still incomplete; the evidence that overwork can damage your health is virtually uncontested.

Exercising the brain through lifelong learning helps keep you mentally sharp as you age. Rudolph Tanzi, Ph.D., professor of neurology at Harvard Medical School, discusses some fascinating medical evidence in *Decoding Darkness: The Search for the Genetic Causes of Alzheimer's Disease.* The evidence suggests that dementia probably results from losing too many synapses, which are part of the intricate system used by brain cells to transmit information to other parts of the body. Tanzi concludes that the more synapses you develop through participating in intellectually stimulating activities, the more you can "afford" to lose before dementia might occur. According to Dr. Tanzi, playing mental games, working crossword puzzles, playing bridge or chess, and having stimulating conversations are all ways to nurture lifelong learning.

More recent research confirms that, like muscles, the brain must be exercised. According to the Alzheimer's Foundation, older people in good physical health who have more years of education and a higher income and who are employed generally do better in memory performance than other seniors. A 2002 study of 801 older Catholic nuns, priests, and brothers without dementia at enrollment—recruited from forty groups across the United States—concluded that frequent participation in cognitively stimulating activities was associated with a significantly reduced risk of Alzheimer's disease.

Active mental stimulation—exercising your mind—may give you a brain reserve. However, watching television and doing channel surfing probably do nothing to help increase the number of synapses you have in the "bank."

Check Your Emotional Pressure

It's easy to get so busy that we fail to "check in" with ourselves to ask, as we would of a loved one, "How are you—really?" "Are you happy?" "Are you overwhelmed or bored, satisfied or frustrated?"

So give yourself the gift of a "time-out"—at least twenty minutes in length. Check the "pressure" in your emotional wheel by taking a close look at each of your spokes. Which spoke is the shortest? Write in a journal (or jot brief notes to yourself) about what seems to be causing you the most pressure or dissatisfaction. Then make an appointment—this week!—with your spouse or a trusted friend to talk about what you wrote down regarding your emotional wheel. Ask that person to review the four spokes with you and help you come up with at least one thing you can do to add some length to the shortest spoke.

Above all, be gentle with yourself. Highly healthy people don't beat themselves up just because they're not perfect! You'll *never* be perfect, but you can be healthier.

I suspect it's becoming clear to you: the lengths of the spokes and the balance of your wheels can constantly change. In one year your wheel can be fairly balanced—and then, seemingly in the batting of an eye, it can flatten. How you respond to your "flat tire" may determine how your health will turn out down the road.

RELATIONAL BALANCE

Leon was more than a patient—he became a good and trusted friend. But when I met him, he was a mess.

His wife of nearly fifty years had died suddenly. She wasn't only his best friend; she was his only friend. They had moved to Florida to escape the bitterly cold winters of their hometown—and although they found a warm (even hot) environment, they left all of their family and friends.

Leon's life soon became absorbed with caring for his frail wife. They had no friends and never socialized with others. As her condition worsened, so did his. I'd make frequent home visits to see them, and in the back of my mind I wondered who would die first. If she preceded him, I was sure he'd die of a broken heart soon after. He was not open to my suggestions that he do things outside of the home and begin to care for himself as well as for his wife.

She *was* the first to go. At her funeral, I witnessed a man break apart. His grief was palpable. As I continued to visit him from time to time, I observed that he was worsening quickly. He was so lonely.

Leon's relationships with his parents, spouse, children, and extended family had been superb. Although he never did a wheel drawing (I knew Leon before I developed these drawings), I'm convinced those spokes would have been full. But he had outlived them all. Here he was, alone and dying—not from illness but from a totally flat relational wheel.

Then something happened to recharge his batteries, to rejuvenate his health and his will to live, to turn him around physically and emotionally. I had almost given up. His home was so dismal—so dark. I had begun to raise orchids, and I had one that was blooming in a spectacular fashion. I decided to give it to Leon—to try to bring some "color" into his life.

The day I went out to our greenhouse to get the orchid, I came upon a small kitten just outside the greenhouse. I had no idea how she got there. I picked up the kitten and the orchid, put them in my pickup truck, and drove to Makinson's Hardware Store in downtown Kissimmee to pick up supplies to use in caring for both kitten and orchid, and then headed to Leon's.

When he saw my gifts, the biggest smile spread over his face—the first ear-to-ear grin I'd seen on him in quite some time—but not the last.

The kitten made him an instant hit in the trailer park. It seemed to become what he would later call "a babe magnet" (referring to the widows who just happened to "drop by" to see how the kitten was doing).

The orchid seemed to ignite his interests and creativity. He began visiting local orchid growers and then began taking classes in orchid care. His circle of friends grew—as did his confidence, his radiance, and his health. It was as if he bloomed with each orchid. He loved bringing orchids to the office to show off to my staff and me.

Leon lived for another ten years. And in those ten years he *really* lived. He was, for me, living proof of the value of relationships, interests, hobbies, and pets, not only in terms of nurturing good health but also in restoring declining health. Without these things, I have no doubt I would have attended Leon's funeral many, many years earlier—and with much less joy than when he went to be with the Lord at almost eighty-five years of age.

Check the Rust on Your Trust

On a scale of 1 to 7 (1 = extremely distrustful; 4 = sometimes trusting, sometimes not; 7 = extremely trusting), how much trust do you think you have in other human beings? (Remember, be honest!) Carefully consider why you answered the way you did. If you want your relational wheel to be full and balanced, you'll need to have clarity on why it may *not* be. Now make a list of the top five "safest" relationships in your life. Then make a list of the top five relationships that cause you distress of any kind. With these lists in front of you, talk them over with the Creator who loves you. Pour out your heart— your gratitude, your sadness, your joy, your fear. Sit quietly for a while, tuning your inner ear to the voice of divine wisdom. Consider reading some of the best prose about love ever written—1 Corinthians 13 in the Bible. Then write down at least *one* thought about how you might deal more effectively with a relationship that is causing distress or imbalance. Finally, if someone you love and trust is close by, give him or her a hug!

SPIRITUAL BALANCE

Jimmy was self-absorbed—and miserable. Oh, it was hard to tell from the outside. He was a millionaire, had a gorgeous wife and kids, drove the best cars, and lived in a beautiful house on the lake. Physically, emotionally, and relationally he seemed balanced and healthy—but his spiritual wheel was flat.

Jimmy didn't recognize it for quite some time. He was convinced that he didn't need God—that everything was just fine, thank you. Then it began. Those middle-age doubts. During a morning workout we were sharing he wondered out loud, "What's the real meaning of life?" As we talked he expressed doubt that life has a purpose. He felt clueless about whether there is anything after life on this earth. It turned out that Jimmy was beginning one of the most important searches of his life—the search for spiritual significance.

"Jim," I asked, "how would you like to get together once a week and take a look at what the Bible has to say about these questions?"

Somewhat to my surprise, he enthusiastically agreed. "Never really looked at the Bible. Just thought it was an old dusty book. But my grandpa lived by its every word. I've always wanted to take a look inside."

Although I'm not a trained theologian, I had spent time studying what the Bible has to say about the things Jimmy wondered about: family life, business, money, success, and the meaning of life. Jimmy was a voracious learner, and our discussions were fun and wide-ranging.

Based on his reading and study, Jimmy decided that he wanted to begin a personal relationship with God. I vividly remember the moment he bowed his head in prayer to admit to God all of his wrongdoing and dubious motives and simply asked God to come into his life and make him the kind of person his Creator wanted him to be.

Jimmy's spiritual spokes soon lengthened dramatically. He spent time every day in Bible study and prayer. We continued meeting weekly to learn more and more about our God and his words in the Bible. Jimmy and his family found a church and became active in it. Watching his spiritual growth was like watching a small child in a candy store.

Then an amazing thing happened. Jimmy began sharing his spiritual journey with his friends and colleagues who had "flat" spiritual wheels like he'd once had. He didn't push his faith on them; he just asked questions and found others who, like himself, were hungry to learn more about God and his principles for becoming highly healthy in all four wheels. Over time, as Jimmy's spiritual wheel was filled, all of his other health wheels became more balanced. What a transformation—not only in Jimmy but also in his family and eventually in several of his friends!

Scrutinize Your Spiritual Spokes

Look carefully at your spiritual spokes, noting which ones need the most "lengthening." Pay attention to how you feel about each of these spokes. Does reviewing any (or all of them) make you uncomfortable, excited, anxious, motivated? Ask yourself why. Then write down an answer to this simple question: "What is your concept of God right now?" You may come up with an answer quickly and easily, or you may feel stumped for a while. But resolve to put down your answer in writing and date it. Don't write down what you think you *should* feel or believe; be absolutely authentic about what is true for you at this very moment. Then as you move through the rest of the book—especially chapter 8—revisit your answer and see if it is changing over time. Growing spiritually is an exciting adventure. Mark your starting point, and watch what God does as you journey down the road toward becoming more highly healthy.

KEEPING YOUR BALANCE

How many people have I met who have all four wheels perfectly balanced? *None.* Not a single one.

The important thing to remember is that we were all created differently. We share a common need to balance the different parts of our life; many of our needs are, in fact, the same. But we were all designed by our Creator to have our needs met uniquely and differently.

Maintaining a healthy balance is a lifelong and life-enhancing task.

CHAPTER FOUR

Be Proactive in Preventing Disease

The Essential of Self-Care

It may seem obvious, but the secret to becoming and staying highly healthy is to prevent "dis-ease" in body, in mind, in spirit, and in relationships—as much as is possible. As a family physician, I rarely saw a patient with a previously preventable medical problem who didn't wish he or she had done more—expended more time and effort—to prevent the problem that was now troubling him or her.

I spent my first year of medical practice in the Smoky Mountains of rural western North Carolina. There I had the privilege of caring for a number of patients who were in their nineties—and several who were over one hundred years old. Caring for these men and women taught me much about what it means to be a highly healthy person.

Margaret had just turned ninety when we first met. "I'm tired of traveling all the way to Sylva to see the internist," she told me during our first appointment. "And," she added, "my doctor over there is so old. I'm afraid he's not going to be around much longer!"

"How old is he?" I asked.

She giggled, putting her hand over her mouth, blushing. "Oh, honey, he's barely sixty. He just doesn't know how to live very well. And I think he's working himself into an early grave! If he had just listened to me."

I smiled to myself. Here was a woman thirty years older than her physician, predicting his death. Barely one month later, I saw his obituary in the newspaper.

Margaret had my attention, and over the next four years I listened and she taught. Hardly a visit went by where she didn't share her wisdom. Here are some of what my office staff called "Margaretisms":

- When asked why she always seemed so up, never moody or down, even when an illness flared, she exclaimed, "I'm too blessed to be stressed or depressed!"
- When talking about a local politician who had been accused of an ethical indiscretion, she quipped, "Forbidden fruits create many jams."
- She told me that she exercised twice as much as most people: "Every day I walk an hour along Deep Creek and I walk twenty-four hours with the Lord."

One afternoon I noticed my nurse, Beth, doubled over in laughter as Margaret was leaving the office. I had prescribed a mild medication to help her with occasional insomnia. She also was taking a laxative sporadically for bouts of constipation. She had pointed out to Beth, "Honey, whatever else you do, never, never, under any circumstances, have a patient take a sleeping pill and a laxative on the same night." Then she took off out the door to conquer the world.

Margaret had a number of physical and mental ailments, but minor "mechanical" problems aren't too noticeable in an "older vehicle" that has been well cared for and is otherwise running efficiently. And Margaret was running efficiently.

Margaret had a number of similarities with her long-lived friends, as well as with other elderly folks from various cultures who, because of their longevity, have been studied. Leonard W. Poon, the lead researcher in one of the largest studies of centenarians ever conducted, reported that centenarians find meaning in life's trials and respond effectively to problems. They're not "wallowers." Margaret was no wallower!

Some of the longest long-lived groups of people in the world are said to be among the Georgians of the Caucasus Mountains in southern Russia, the Vilcabamba Indians of the Ecuadorian Andes, the people of the Hunza Valley in Kashmir, and residents of Okinawa, Japan. Not only are they long-lived, with significant numbers of individuals exceeding one hundred years of age, but medical studies also accent the high quality of life of most of the centenarians in these cultures. As scientists have tried to identify common elements, they've reported the following characteristics of these non-American centenarians:

- *They exercise regularly and consistently.* Walking and other forms of active exercise are part of their everyday lives.
- *They avoid highly processed foods.* In fact, virtually none of their food is highly processed, as are many of our junk foods and fast foods here in the United States.
- *They eat a nutritious diet.* They don't overeat, and their diet is high in fiber, whole grains, nuts, and "good" fats (and in some cultures, yogurt or soy) and low in calories, salt, saturated fats, and refined sugars. Health-enhancing fish also is an important staple of the diet in some of these cultures.
- *They drink lots of water.* In most of these cultures, the water is usually from wells or mountain streams and has a high mineral content.
- *They consume plenty of fresh fruits and vegetables.*
- *They avoid loneliness.* Relationships within their communities with neighbors, family, and friends are vital.
- *They practice and enjoy regular sex*—usually with their spouse, who is their longtime partner in a mutually monogamous relationship, even after the age of one hundred.
- *They live with and depend on their extended families,* who offer cradle-to-grave security and support. The concept of a nursing home is not only unheard-of, it would not be tolerated.
- *They seldom use alcohol or tobacco products.*
- *They intensely respect their elders.* And when they become elderly, they enjoy the admiration, honor, esteem, and affection of their families and of society.
- *They lead active, fruitful lives well into their second century.* There is no retirement. They may slow down a bit, but they never stop.
- *They emphasize relationships and harmony over the pursuit of wealth or success.* Many of these people would be considered poor by Western standards. Yet they consider themselves wealthy and satisfied.

A group of more than one hundred centenarians living within an eight-town radius of Boston, Massachusetts, were the subjects of a study initiated in 1994. These are some of the important characteristics they share:

- Significant obesity is rare.
- Smoking history is extremely rare.
- They score low in a type of personality testing that measures neuroticism (based on a preliminary study). A lack of neuroticism translates into not dwelling on problems and therefore managing stress well.
- They have a history of showing signs of aging very slowly and markedly delaying or even escaping age-associated diseases, such as heart attack, stroke, cancer, diabetes, and Alzheimer's disease.

- Ninety percent of the centenarians studied are functionally independent for the vast majority of their lives—up until the average age of ninety-two years. Rather than the incorrect perception that the older you become, the sicker you get, these centenarians teach us that the healthier you've been, the older you get.
- Many centenarian women have a history of bearing children after the age of thirty-five and even forty. A woman who gives birth after the age of forty has a four times greater chance of living to one hundred than women who do not. It's probably not the act of bearing a child in one's forties that promotes long life, but doing so may be an indicator that the woman's reproductive system is aging slowly and that the rest of her body is just as healthy.
- At least 50 percent have close relatives and/or grandparents who lived to a very old age, and many have exceptionally old siblings. Male siblings of centenarians have an eleven times greater chance of reaching age ninety-seven than other men born around the same time, and female siblings have an eight and a half times greater chance of achieving age one hundred than other females born around the same time.
- Many children of these centenarians (age range of sixty-five to eighty-two) appear to be following in their parents' footsteps.

The codirectors of this New England Centenarian Study (NECS)—Thomas Perls, M.D., M.P.H., and Margery Hutter Silver, Ed.D.—have published their observations in the medical literature and in a popular book titled *Living to 100: Lessons in Living to Your Maximum Potential at Any Age.*

I think the most reassuring of the NECS findings is that while the centenarians share certain characteristics, they are not all alike. In fact, they have a wide range of different characteristics—their ethnicity, religion, level of education (no formal schooling to postgraduate study), socioeconomic status (very poor to very rich), dietary patterns (strictly vegetarian to extremely rich in saturated fats), and exercise (none to daily).

IT'S MORE THAN GOOD GENES

Researchers tell us that the odds of living to one hundred years of age are increasing every year. There are already many thousands of centenarians alive today, and at least half of them are well enough to live independently. There are about 50,000 people over the age of one hundred in the United States alone—almost three times as many as there were in 1980.

Are they just lucky in the "good genes" department? Or is their health due to the way they live? While scientists continue to debate the factors that are most likely to assist us in becoming centenarians, most now say that long life is *not just* a result of good genes. Genes are important, but even more important are the decisions we make about a variety of daily lifestyle issues—eating, sleeping, diet, exercise, work, leisure, and our relationships. Some experts believe that as much as 80 percent of what controls how long you or I will live is related to our lifestyle choices, not our genes. We'll be exploring these factors—captured by the "ten essentials"—in depth throughout the book.

Quickly Evaluate Your Lifestyle

Look back and study the two lists above that describe characteristics of people who live to be one hundred years old. List at least one thing about your lifestyle that you believe is already working in your favor. Then list all the "room for improvement" points so you'll have them as a starting point on your journey toward becoming more proactive about your health.

EXPOSING THE TRUTH ABOUT PREVENTABLE DEATHS

Since the terrorist attacks on September 11, 2001, and the subsequent bioterrorist attacks with anthrax bacteria spores, people are appropriately concerned about the threat of future attacks to their health and safety. However, the average American is much more likely to die from a shark attack or a lightning strike than from an anthrax infection. And you are one hundred times more likely to die from influenza than from the West Nile virus—and flu deaths are uncommon. The reality is that about two million Americans die each year—and many of these deaths could be prevented. In 2000, the leading causes of death in the United States were

1. heart disease (709,894, translating to about 29.5 percent of all deaths—or about 1 in every 3.4 deaths).
2. cancer (551,833, about 23 percent of all deaths—or 1 in every 4 deaths).
3. stroke (166,028, about 7 percent of all deaths—or 1 in every 14 deaths). Note that cardiovascular diseases (which include heart disease and stroke), make up the number one and number three killers

in the U.S.—about 36.4 percent of all deaths, or about 1 in every 2.7 deaths).

4. chronic lower respiratory disease (123,550, about 5 percent of all deaths—or about 1 in every 20 deaths).
5. accidents (93,592, about 3.9 percent—or about 1 in 25 deaths).
6. diabetes (68,662, about 2.8 percent—or about 1 in every 36 deaths).
7. pneumonia and influenza (67,024, about 2.8 percent—or about 1 in every 36 deaths).
8. Alzheimer's disease (49,044, about 2 percent—or about 1 in every 50 deaths).
9. kidney disease (37,672, 1.6 percent—or about 1 in every 60 deaths).
10. septicemia, or infections of the blood (31,613, about 1.3 percent—or about 1 in every 75 deaths).

Many women believe that breast cancer is their main health concern when, in fact, this disease is far down the list. The latest statistics from the American Heart Association show that 512,914 women died in 1999 from a largely preventable group of conditions—high blood pressure and coronary artery disease (including heart attack and angina, stroke, congenital cardiovascular defects, and congestive heart failure). According to the Centers for Disease Control, 41,528 women died from breast cancer in 1999. For every woman who dies from breast cancer, almost nine die from a heart attack and more than two die from a stroke.

DECEPTIVE ADVICE AND ADS

Experts estimate that more than half of the deaths in America each year may well have been preventable. Of these preventable deaths, cigarette smoking causes half, and one-fifth are the result of alcohol addiction. The solution in these cases seems to be simple: Don't smoke, and don't drink. But for many it's not that simple. Starting is easy; stopping is hard. The teens now gathered in small groups—each person with a cigarette in hand—represent the next generation, which, barring a dramatic change, will face these same statistics on preventable deaths forty years from now.

What is feeding this trend? What are we doing as a society to educate ourselves about making wise choices with regard to our health? Why aren't the real dangers from things such as smoking better understood and heeded? Why is so much good information ignored?

Much of what is presented in magazines and newspapers and on television and radio regarding critical health information is too often inaccurate or misleading. We are bombarded with advice—to the point where we can no longer sort it out, and we tend to ignore much of it.

In 1992, Elizabeth M. Whelan, Sc.D., M.P.H., reviewed two consecutive months of articles (July and August) in the ten most popular women's magazines *(Redbook, Glamour, New Woman, Cosmopolitan, Vanity Fair, Self, Family Circle, Mademoiselle, McCall's,* and *Harper's Bazaar).* She found that the articles focused not on the most common detrimental lifestyle factors but on the "alleged ill effects of trace level chemicals and other hypothetical causes."

For example, *Redbook* and *Glamour* reported on levels of methyl mercury and PCBs in fish, which could supposedly cause cancer. *Glamour* warned readers that eating imported fresh fruit could be hazardous to their health because the surface of the fruit might be contaminated with bacteria. According to Dr. Whelan, other publications raised red flags about the dangers of salt; cancer-causing substances in grilled meat; electromagnetic fields emanating from refrigerators, stoves, and alarm clocks (to reduce our risk of cancer, *Family Circle* cautioned us to keep dial-face clocks five feet and digitals three feet from our beds—although there is no compelling medical evidence to support this recommendation); radiation emissions from computers; breast implants; toilet seats and hot tubs; lead wrappers on wine bottles and in dinnerware; contaminants in recycled food containers; high-intensity halogen lights (*Harper's Bazaar* recommended we use a plastic cover to block out potentially harmful ultraviolet rays—once again with no evidence to support such an expense); thrill rides at amusement parks; and even the weather.

Dr. Whelan asked, "So what type of advice do the magazines offer women on how to stay healthy?" Here is a sampling: eat lots of broccoli to ward off cancer *(Redbook)*; take vitamins E and C and beta carotene to protect against heart disease and cancer *(Glamour)*; eat garlic to fight colds and flu *(McCall's)*; get a pet to lower blood pressure and cholesterol *(Self)*; and eat active-culture yogurt to live longer *(Harper's Bazaar).*

Dr. Whelan contends that much of the health advice presented in these articles was not based on solid scientific evidence, and was in fact a distortion of scientific reality. She also contends that cigarette advertising revenue, in particular, "places a chill on the free discussion of the dangers of smoking, a topic only rarely touched upon by these publications." One issue of *New Woman* expressed outrage about breast implants while carrying twenty-three cigarette ads. An editorial in *Cosmopolitan*—surrounded by cigarette ads—demanded that more funding be supplied for research on women's health issues, while failing to note that lung cancer causes more deaths among American women than does breast cancer.

Dr. Whelan concludes, "If historians ever wonder about the underlying causes of inverted health priorities that characterize our nation's public health policies today—policies which draw attention to the alleged dangers of everything from apples to bacon to electric blankets, yet ignore the significance of nearly $4 billion in advertisements for the leading cause of death—they need look no further than the magazines at today's newsstands."

Although these findings are ten years old, we still see these types of articles. In fact, a 1998 article observed, "Tobacco companies have long held a special spot in their hearts for women, courting them aggressively. Tactics include everything from marketing slim cigarettes with the now-famous slogan 'You've come a long way, baby' to underwriting women's political events."

Things are no better at the movie theaters. This same article tells us that "Hollywood is playing its part, too, as more actors and actresses light up in movies." Take the movie *Basic Instinct,* for example, which seems to glamorize smoking. Joe Eszterhas, screenwriter for that movie and more than a dozen others (including *Flashdance* and *Showgirls*) was diagnosed with throat cancer after a lifetime of smoking. In an op-ed piece in *The New York Times,* Eszterhas urged Hollywood to stop glamorizing cigarette use the way he once did. He wrote, "I have been an accomplice to the murders of untold numbers of human beings. I am admitting this only because I have made a deal with God. 'Spare me,' I said, 'and I will try to stop others from committing the same crimes I did.'" The writer concluded, "My hands are bloody; so are Hollywood's."

IT'S YOUR CHOICE

In large measure you determine your own destiny with regard to becoming and remaining a highly healthy person. Family history and genetics play a role, to be sure, but it is increasingly obvious that our lifestyle decisions play a much larger role. The Bible teaches that it is our sacred duty to be proactive about our own self-care. God considers the human body, which he designed, to be a "temple": "Don't you know that you yourselves are God's temple and that God's Spirit lives in you?... God's temple is sacred, and you are that temple."

Learning to avoid the allure of the ever-so-slick Madison Avenue advertising agencies is important, but becoming educated about the facts and what *you* can do to become more highly healthy is critical.

So let's get to work. Pull out the diagram of your four health wheels and their spokes. How round is your physical health wheel? Is it small, or is it large? Which spokes most need your attention? The self-assessments sprinkled throughout the remainder of this chapter can help you determine where you need to place your focus as you work toward preventing the most common physical diseases.

THE TEN COMMANDMENTS OF PREVENTIVE MEDICINE

Below is a list of the top ten rules I've long suggested to my patients and to my radio and television audiences. These "Ten Commandments" target exclusively the physical wheel. I suspect we could identify several more commandments related to preventing disease, but these are an excellent start. You may not find a lot of surprises here—but the real questions are these: Which of these rules do you need to begin to follow? When do you plan to start? What strategies will ensure your success? By beginning with a single step and then continuing to improve on a day-to-day basis, you'll be on your way to becoming a highly healthy person.

1. See a Primary Care Physician for Preventive Maintenance and Care

I broke down and purchased a car a few years ago. My 1979 pickup truck had finally died. It had been quite some time since I had purchased a vehicle, and it was a pleasant surprise to find that the newer cars come equipped with a maintenance schedule. When I looked at it, I was reminded of the preventive medicine schedules I used in my practice. Most preventive medicine experts recommend a schedule by which adults and children should have certain types of preventive care—such as screening tests and immunizations. The timing of these services depends on your body's "model" and "mileage" (that is, your gender and age).

Unfortunately, most adults and many children and adolescents have fallen way behind on their maintenance schedules. For example, colon cancer screening is recommended for everyone (male and female) over the age of fifty—but 59 percent in this age group have not been tested. Everyone over the age of sixty-five should receive a single immunization against pneumococcal pneumonia and an annual flu shot—but more than a third of all Americans in this age group didn't get a flu shot in 2001, and more than 60 percent have never received the potentially life-saving pneumonia vaccine. According to the latest statistics available (in 2000) these two illnesses—influenza and pneumonia—were the seventh-leading cause of death in the U.S.—prematurely taking the lives of more than 67,000 people.

If you haven't been taking routine care of your body, resolve to make an appointment with your doctor this year to find out which preventive services are recommended for your age and gender. And then follow up by getting the recommended tests and immunizations.

Time to Get Shot

The National Network for Immunization Information is sponsored by several medical professional societies. You can visit this online information center and find up-to-date immunization schedules for different age groups at my Website at www.highly healthy.net. There you can access the site(s) that apply to you and your children and make sure you're up-to-date on your immunizations. If you're not, call your doctor's office to schedule an appointment.

2. Avoid or Reduce Obesity

Obesity is now an epidemic in America. Over 70 percent of the adults in the U.S. in 2001 were either overweight or obese—with more than 50 percent being overweight and at least 22 percent being obese (meaning they weigh at least 30 percent more than they should). The proportion of the population that is overweight has gone up at least 30 percent over the last thirty years. Excess weight is associated with increased risk of heart disease, diabetes, high blood pressure, stroke, arthritis, gallbladder disease, depression, fatigue, poor work performance, sleep disturbances, and several forms of cancer—and that's only a sampling of the many diseases associated with being overweight.

According to the *Journal of the American Medical Association,* in 1999 nearly 900 people died every day from weight-related illnesses, which added up to almost 325,000 deaths a year—more than the number killed annually by pneumonia, motor vehicle accidents, and airline crashes combined, and three-fourths as many as the 430,000 who die yearly from tobacco-related conditions. Health care costs for weight-related illnesses total an estimated $117 billion annually.

Clearly both adults and children could eat better. The surgeon general has recommended that restaurants and fast-food establishments—where Americans spend about 40 percent of their food budget—should offer more nutrition information. The report suggests that employers include weight management and physical activity counseling in their health insurance coverage and allow employees time to exercise. Obesity should also be classified as a disease to encourage insurance companies to reimburse for weight control expenses, the report concludes.

We're all aware that there are more diet plans available in bookstores than the average person could read in a lifetime. And the diet gurus are constantly squabbling over why their diet plan works and no one else's does. All trustworthy nutrition scientists, however, agree that the keys to good nutrition include variety, moderation, and balance. There are very few foods that can always be considered good or bad, but there certainly are good and bad nutrition plans—and fad diets.

If you are overweight and are interested in reasonable approaches to nutrition, invest in a family consultation with a registered dietician or find a nearby Weight Watchers group. In the early 1990s, Barb and I improved our dietary habits and began a regular program of walking. Over the course of time I've been able to take off twenty-five pounds and keep it off. If you find that you're overweight and unable to keep weight off, make an appointment with your physician or a weight-loss specialist to discuss your options. Take action—today—for a healthier future. To put it simply, to help reduce excess weight and to maintain a healthy weight, eat a balanced diet, reduce your total calorie intake, eat less fat, and exercise regularly.

3. Exercise Regularly—with Caution

As you probably are well aware, dietary and nutrition changes, in and of themselves, almost never translate to significant weight loss. In order to achieve and maintain an ideal body weight and to become a highly healthy person, you simply *must* exercise. People who exercise frequently, even if it's weeding in the garden or walking around the block, enjoy better overall health—physically and emotionally. Not only that, exercise may also assist you in controlling what you eat. In other words, exercise and good nutrition can help each other help you.

People who exercise at least three hours a week tend to eat a more balanced and a healthier diet, one research study found. The researchers gave several reasons for their findings:

- *People who exercise think twice before overindulging.* When I would explain to my patients that eating the average meal at a fast-food restaurant would require a one- to two-hour walk to work off the calories, they sometimes found it easier to "just say no."
- *The more you exercise, the more you can eat.* Recent research from the U.S. Department of Agriculture has shown that the vast majority of people (though not all) can lose weight if they simply consume fewer than 1,500 calories per day. If you're exercising regularly, then you could take in 1,700 to 1,800 calories a day and achieve the same effect.

If you eat fewer than 1,500 calories a day *and* exercise daily, then you will almost certainly lose weight and keep it off.

• *Exercise makes you feel healthier than eating does.* Once people begin to eat better and exercise daily, they notice remarkably bad feelings when they revert to old habits. Most of my patients who began to exercise boasted of improved skin health, increased stamina and work performance, increased energy, more restful sleep, and an improved sex life. You won't get that from a fad diet! My daughter, Kate, cut out all beverages except for tea and water while in college. "Dad," she told me, "I can't believe how *sweet* soft drinks taste now." Many people will notice that desserts or red meats make them feel sluggish after they've stopped consuming them for a period of time.

Regular exercise will help you control your weight, improve your overall health, and reduce your risk of such medical problems as diabetes, heart disease, and osteoporosis. According to the Centers for Disease Control, we should exercise for at least thirty minutes five days per week. The CDC reports that fewer than one-third of all Americans exercise this much. "This is probably the most sedentary generation of people in the history of the world," America's surgeon general declared in 2001. The National Academy of Sciences' Institute of Medicine issued a report in September 2002 containing this recommendation: "To maintain cardiovascular health at a maximal level, regardless of weight, adults and children also should spend a total of at least one hour each day in moderately intense physical activity."

It is clear from the medical studies that *any* exercise is better than none. Your fitness level, which can be determined by a cardiac stress test, may be the single best predictor of your risk of dying prematurely—whether or not you have a diagnosed heart disease, suggests an extensive study of more than 6,000 men over the course of more than six years. Besides predicting the presence of heart disease, a cardiac stress test evaluates your fitness—and routinely reports this as an exercise capacity or fitness level (which the doctors call aerobic capacity). This level is expressed in units called METS—metabolic equivalents. In this study, men with a fitness level of five METS or fewer had twice the chance of dying as people with a METS level of eight or more—whether they had heart disease or not. In other words, exercise and aerobic fitness are strongly associated with a longer and more highly healthy life. In the past, the cardiac stress test was used primarily for testing the level of disease of the heart. However, this study shows that this exercise test can now be used to test wellness and to predict overall health risk.

Many who begin to exercise develop a common problem: They quit! And pretty quickly, according to sports psychologist William F. Morgan of the University of Wisconsin-Madison. Within six to eight weeks, 50 percent have quit exercising; another 25 percent quit by the end of one year. His research shows that the approach of joining a health club, doing weight training, running, and the like doesn't motivate most people. He believes that people do not need exercise *programs* as much as they just need physical activity that is part of their daily lives and has some sense of purpose. Dr. Morgan notes that one of the best exercise machines available is the family dog—it has to go on its daily walk, with owner in tow. Similarly, people who walk to work (by parking a considerable distance from the building) and who take the stairs (rather than the elevator) will get healthful activity, even though they may not think of it as exercise.

Setting a goal when exercising—to lose weight, to avoid weakening of the bones, to add a bit to one's life span—can impart much personal meaning to physical activity. However, the challenge is to overcome the initial tedium and discomfort in order to get to the point where the benefits kick in. The best thing to do? Minimize the discomfort and accentuate the enjoyment of the activity.

I recommend that you find an activity you like and that you do it with a person you like, and then that you keep doing it regularly until it becomes a habit. Getting support from a small group of friends or colleagues can provide the meaning that will be transformed into motivation to continue exercising. Beginning exercisers are less likely to drop out if they think they will lose face in their group or will let down other members by not showing up. Accountability counts!

Some people do best with a personal trainer. My wife, Barb, and several of her friends hired a personal trainer to work with them at a gym three days a week. The trainer helped them keep their goals positive and aligned with reality. She taught them wise and valuable workout techniques that matched their physiques and personalities. The trainer helped build their confidence as a group by targeting small but achievable increases and discouraging lofty goals that would have been tough to achieve. Splitting the cost with several others also made it very affordable!

Time to Move

Follow these steps to success in beginning and then continuing to exercise as a natural part of your lifestyle:

- Get started—don't delay.
- Pick a form (or forms) of exercise that you enjoy. (Or at the very least, do something else that you enjoy as you exercise. Walking on a treadmill may become more enjoyable if you can read while walking.)
- Exercise with a partner or a group.

Be sure to take all the safety precautions recommended for the activities you choose. Wearing a helmet while cycling, skiing, or skating can reduce your risk of head injury by 85 percent. Other safety equipment (such as knee pads and wrist guards) also reduces your risk of injury when you are roller-blading.

Although exercise is beneficial for almost everyone, some people need to consult a doctor to find out what level and types of physical activities are safe for them. This precaution is especially important for pregnant women, people who have a medical condition that might be aggravated by exercise (such as diabetes, arthritis, or angina), and people who are taking any type of medication (especially medicines for high blood pressure or heart disease).

4. Consider the Benefits of a Lifelong Monogamous Marriage Relationship

Married people are, in general, more highly healthy than singles or those who live together without the commitment of marriage. Married people live longer and generally are more emotionally and physically healthy than the unmarried. That's the finding of more than 130 studies conducted from the 1930s to the present. Simply put, marriage offers important health benefits to individuals and society that no other relational status can match.

Marriage—to the extent that both the husband and wife are monogamous—also can protect a man and a woman from sexually transmitted infections (STIs), which have become epidemic in the United States. Every day, 8,000 teenagers contract an STI—about three million teenagers per year! Of the approximately 15.3 million new cases of STIs that occur annually in the United States, one in four of the victims is younger than twenty.

Sexually transmitted infections accounted for five of the ten most common reportable infectious diseases in this country in 1999 (the most recent year for which data was available): chlamydia (#1), gonorrhea (#2), AIDS (#3), hepatitis B (#9), and syphilis (#10). The Centers for Disease Control (CDC) does not collect data on other common sexually transmitted diseases, such as herpes and human papillomavirus (HPV). However, a study published in the *New England Journal of Medicine* estimated that 20 percent of all Americans age twelve and over are infected with genital herpes. And HPV is the most prevalent viral STI—having been shown to be present in as many as 60 percent of the sexually active population that has more than one sex partner. HPV causes over 90 percent of cancer and precancer of the cervix and is associated with cancer of the penis and prostate. Once you get one of the STIs caused by a virus, you can have it for life, and STIs, like HPV, can be spread by intimate touching (not just by sexual intercourse)—and can be contracted with the *first* contact. That's why some experts say, "When you have sex with someone, you are instantly having sex with everyone that he or she has ever had sex with."

Why have sexually transmitted infections become so common? Put simply, it's because nonmarital sexual activity is epidemic. I'd suggest another possible reason—what I call the "safe sex" myth. While experts at the CDC tell us that adolescents and adults often don't use condoms consistently or correctly, one might ask if this is really the answer? The CDC data shows, for example, that only 57 percent of high school students reported using a condom the last time they had intercourse. What's more, a 2001 CDC report showed that condoms were proven to be effective only in reducing the risk of HIV/AIDS and gonorrhea in men; for all other STIs, the evidence is insufficient to declare that condoms are effective.

Even when used consistently and correctly, however, both contraceptives and condoms can fail—and even a small failure rate per use will slowly increase the risk of an STI over time. It's also important to remember that condoms can't protect sexually active persons from those STIs that are transmitted by skin-to-skin contact (rather than by body fluids). These include genital herpes and the dangerous HPV. And condoms never protect the hearts—the emotions and spirits—of people.

When it comes to incurable and potentially fatal viral infections such as AIDS, hepatitis B, and hepatitis C, experts say that the following can reduce your risk:

- Avoid tattoos and body piercing of any kind (except earrings).
- Never use (or allow anyone else to use) a nonsterile needle to inject anything into your body.
- Don't use illicit drugs. (Snorting cocaine has now been associated with hepatitis C.)
- Either abstain from sex or have sex only in marriage and a mutually monogamous lifelong relationship. If you choose to have multiple sex partners (or your partner chooses to do so), then you run a very high risk of contracting a sexually transmitted infection.

Sexual abstinence until marriage and fidelity after marriage clearly reduce your risk for these dangerous forms of preventable—but often untreatable—infections. The bottom line is that the only "safe sex" physically, emotionally, and spiritually is to wait until marriage—and increasingly our young people are hearing and heeding this message. In 2001, 54 percent of high school seniors were virgins—and the percent continues to increase each year.

5. Protect Your Dental Health

You probably already know that you can help your teeth stay healthy by brushing and flossing, getting regular dental care, using fluoride as recommended by your doctor or dentist, eating balanced meals, and limiting sugary snacks.

Here's something you may not have heard: Infections of the gums, called gingivitis and periodontitis, has been associated with cardiovascular disease—including heart disease and stroke. Individuals with gum disease have increased levels of abnormal bacteria in their gums. These bacteria have been shown to be more likely than other bacteria to enter the bloodstream. Now researchers believe that these bacteria release toxic substances—called endotoxins—that may explain the link between gum infections and cardiovascular disease. A visit to the dental hygienist every six months, therefore, is not only good for your dental health but also may improve your cardiovascular health. Children, too, should learn good dental health practices in order to prevent the onset of periodontal disease later in life.

Mouth injuries also take a toll on our health. More than two million teeth are knocked out every year, many of them from sports-related injuries. Many of these injuries could have been avoided if the participant had worn a mouth protector. If you play a sport where there's a risk of mouth injury, resolve to wear a mouth guard every time you play.

6. Be Careful with Alcohol

If you drink alcoholic beverages, keep your intake minimal. And always be sure to separate drinking and driving. This rule is a no-brainer—never drink and drive. *Never*. But there's an equally important and often forgotten corollary: Never ride as a passenger in a car driven by someone who has been drinking alcohol—*any* alcohol—even *one* drink. *Never*.

According to the latest statistics collected by the United States Department of Transportation's Fatality Analysis Reporting System (FARS), 38.4 percent of all traffic fatalities in the U.S. were alcohol-related. Nearly 16,000 Americans were killed in 1999 in alcohol-related crashes, and more than 327,000 were injured. Although the number of alcohol-related traffic deaths has dropped by about 30 percent since the late 1980s, there's still plenty of room for improvement. There are more than 120 million episodes of impaired driving in the U.S. every year. Every one of these episodes puts lives at risk. So if you plan to drink, make safe transportation arrangements in advance. If no designated driver is available, use mass transit or call a taxi—or call your local police or sheriff department. In most parts of the country, they will be delighted to assist you. These folks have seen far too many people killed in alcohol-related accidents, and they're eager to prevent any more.

Minimal alcohol intake is not a health risk for most nonpregnant adults. If you're middle-aged or older, some studies indicate that it may even benefit your health by reducing your risk of heart disease. In this book, I'll use the phrase *minimal alcohol intake,* although most medical researchers use the phrase *moderate alcohol intake.*

In any case, what is the definition of *minimal* (or *moderate*)? For men age sixty-five and under, the limit is two drinks per twenty-four hours; for men over sixty-five and women of all ages, it's one drink per day. According to the National Institute on Alcohol Abuse and Alcoholism, a drink is generally considered to be 12 ounces of beer, 5 ounces of wine, or 1.5 ounces of 80-proof distilled spirits. Each of these drinks contains roughly the same amount of absolute alcohol—approximately 0.5 ounce, or 12 grams.

Drinking that goes beyond the bounds of this definition is associated with increased risks of injury, liver disease, heart disease, high blood pressure, and several types of cancer. Drinking is responsible for more than 100,000 deaths in the U.S. each year—not to mention untold misery in terms of addiction, family dysfunction, and crime.

7. Don't Smoke

If you don't smoke, don't start. If you do smoke, resolve to quit *this year.* Half of all adults who once smoked cigarettes have kicked the habit. So can you.

Of all of the New Year's resolutions that will be recorded next January 1, cessation of smoking will be, as it is year after year, one of the most common resolutions—right on up there with the standard resolutions to exercise, lose weight, and eat better. Why? Because many people now know that cigarette smoking is the number one cause of preventable deaths in this country.

And yet, a 2000 survey by Partnership for Prevention, a public health advocacy group based in Washington, D.C., using a nationally representative sample of 1,000 American adults, found that when asked, "What do you think are the leading causes of premature death in the United States?" only 23 percent correctly identified cigarette smoking as number one; 60 percent of us believe that the most likely cause of preventable deaths is either a motor vehicle accident, a drug overdose, or a firearm accident. The truth is that these three together make up less than 10 percent of the preventable deaths each year in our country (and less than 4 percent of all deaths).

Commenting on the study, Partnership for Prevention's president Ashley Coffield said, "Americans are confused about what's really killing them." She went on to note that highly publicized issues like violence and AIDS tend to shape the public's consciousness about health hazards.

Tobacco use is costing Americans $50 billion a year in medical expenditures and is responsible for almost 500,000 deaths in the United States each year. More than half of all lifelong smokers die from a smoking-related disease. Most of the others—those who die from other causes—suffer disability as a result of their addiction to tobacco. According to the American Council on Science and Health, "While [many Americans] associate cigarettes primarily with lung cancer, emphysema, and other lung diseases, smoking is also a major cause of cardiovascular disease (including heart disease and stroke), impotence [erectile dysfunction], and cancers of the mouth, tongue, and esophagus. Cigarette smoking also contributes to cervical, colorectal and kidney tumors, blindness, and hearing loss."

So don't let another year go up in smoke. Start your journey to being highly healthy by becoming and staying smoke-free.

No More Butts

Smoking is dangerous. Smoking is not "cool." It's not "glamorous."

If you smoke, jot down your reasons for smoking. Does it make you feel more mature or elegant? Does it make you feel less alone in some way? Do you enjoy it? Does tobacco use make you feel more upbeat and energetic? Consider that all these reasons involve immediate gratification. But once it's over, the only way to get that feeling again is to have another cigarette.

All the reasons not to smoke entail delayed gratification, and when you're addicted to nicotine, that's a very tall order. But you can make the healthy choice.

If you use tobacco, resolve today to stop. Select a "stop day." Try to find a partner who will stop with you. Let your friends, family, and colleagues know the day so that they can encourage you and hold you accountable. Talk to your doctor or pharmacist about nicotine replacement products that could make the withdrawal easier. And then stop! You can do it. Many already have.

For cutting-edge information on how to stop tobacco abuse, I recommend the American Cancer Society. You can get there from my Website at www.highlyhealthy.net.

8. Check Out Alternative Therapies with Your Doctor

At least 40 percent of Americans use some kind of alternative therapy, such as herbal medicine, dietary supplements, massage therapy, chiropractic, or aromatherapy—among many, many others. Some people mistakenly believe that all alternative practices are harmless. In reality, the risk can be extremely high for people with special medical concerns. Many herbs, vitamins, and supplements can interact with certain prescription drugs, foods, and even other herbs or supplements. They can cause bleeding after surgery and can also interact with anesthetic agents to cause problems with surgery itself—including unexpected death!

Some alternative therapies are contraindicated for certain medical conditions. For example, people with Parkinson's disease should never take the herb kava (sometimes called kava kava), because it can worsen their symptoms. People with severe osteoporosis should not receive certain forms of chiropractic treatment because the manipulation could cause a fracture. People who take the herb ginkgo biloba while also taking an anticoagulant drug can develop bleeding problems. The herb St. John's wort, commonly used for mild depression, may render the birth control pill less effective.

Even if an alternative therapy isn't dangerous in and of itself, you can suffer lasting damage if you use it as a substitute for proper medical care. Most alternatives have not been *proven* effective, and many have been shown not to work at all. If your problem turns out to be serious, you could endanger your health—or even your life—by experimenting with unproven therapies instead of seeing a physician promptly.

If you use alternative therapies—*any* alternative therapy—be sure to let *all* your medical doctors know. More than 60 percent of Americans who use alternative methods don't inform their doctors. Always check with your doctor in order to find out whether an alternative practice you'd like to try is safe for you.

Exercise can be a better treatment option for some disorders—not only better than alternative therapies but sometimes even better than prescription medications. This was demonstrated in a survey of more than 46,000 Americans published by *Consumer Reports* in May 2000. A significant number of the men and women who responded to this survey reported that exercise was more effective than natural remedies for allergies, depression, high cholesterol, sleep problems, and respiratory infections. Even more surprising was the survey's findings that exercise worked as well as prescription medications for arthritis, back pain, and prostate problems.

9. Use Automobile Safety Devices Consistently

Here's a simple one for you. Do you (and everyone who gets into your car) buckle your seat belt *every* time you're in the car—no matter how far you're planning to go? Seat belts save more than 10,000 lives a year in the United States. A survey in 2001 showed that 70 percent of all Americans now buckle up—a 12 percent increase since 1994. While that's good, it could be better. According to Buckle Up America (a national campaign to increase the proper use of seat belts and child safety seats), "Seat belts are a priority. Every hour someone dies in America simply because they didn't buckle up. Failure to wear a seat belt contributes to more fatalities than any other single traffic safety-related behavior."

This year, resolve that everyone in your car will be buckled into the proper restraint before the car moves. That means seat belts for adults, booster seats (in the rear seat) for older children, and properly installed safety seats (in the rear seat) for small children and infants.

10. Install and Maintain Smoke Detectors and Carbon Monoxide Detectors

Smoke detectors save lives. According to the American Academy of Pediatrics, in 1998 there were more than 380,000 residential fires, resulting in nearly 20,000 deaths. For persons of all ages, fires and burns are the fourth most common cause of unintentional injury-related death—after motor vehicles, falls, and poisoning—causing more than 4,000 deaths annually. Eighty percent of all fire deaths take place in residences that don't have operational smoke detectors. Smoke detectors are your best protection against death or injury in a nighttime fire in your home, but they won't protect you if they don't work properly or if the battery is dead or has been removed. The American Red Cross recommends that you test your smoke detectors once a month, replace the batteries at least once a year, and replace the detectors themselves every ten years.

You could also invest in a carbon monoxide detector. Carbon monoxide is a colorless, tasteless, odorless gas that can kill you while you sleep. If your house is heated by gas, most experts recommend that you install a carbon monoxide detector. You can even buy detectors now that will detect both smoke and carbon monoxide.

Plan at least two escape routes from every room in your home, making sure that all family members know how to use them in case of fire or other emergency.

ASSESSING YOUR PHYSICAL HEALTH WHEEL ON THE INTERNET

Scientifically valid health and wellness assessments are typically quite expensive and surprisingly hard to find. With the advent of the Internet, however, many of these somewhat complicated, sophisticated, and expensive tools are now available to you at no cost. When you access these tools on the Internet, they may look almost simplistic. They are often easy-to-take self-assessments. But the software programs used to design them are highly complex. Each answer you generate is plugged in by the computer program to a long and complex mathematical formula based on thousands of bits of data from scientific studies. If I tried to accomplish the same thing in print, you'd never get through it all.

As a result, I'm eager to point out what is available on the Internet. The health assessments I'm recommending are not 100 percent accurate for every person who uses them, but as basic screening instruments, they'll help you begin to sort out the truth about your health. I believe that highly healthy people *must* learn how to make use of the Internet. In fact, I am convinced, and I hope to convince you, that highly healthy people of the twenty-first century *will* use the Internet—and use it often.

If you don't have access to the Internet in your home, or you don't yet know how to use a Web browser or even a computer, don't fret. Most likely you have a friend or relative who has Internet access. Ask someone to help you—almost any teenager can help! If you don't know anyone who has Internet access, then help is probably as close as your nearest public library. More and more educational and business establishments are wired for Internet access, and typically you can use their equipment at little or no cost.

Here's an example of how an Internet health assessment can work. Back in 1994 I auditioned for my first job as a medical journalist—hosting a live, call-in TV show *(Ask the Family Doctor)* on America's Health Network.

One of the calls that day was from Larry. His question: "What can I do about my fatigue? I'm *always* tired."

He seemed short of breath and wheezy just asking the question. Obviously, I had to ask him a few questions in order to accurately assess his situation. I soon learned this: Although Larry was a young man, he smoked, never exercised, worked in a high-stress environment, had a terrible diet, and was obese. His blood pressure, blood sugar, and cholesterol levels were all high—yet he had refused his doctor's recommendation to change his lifestyle or, if not, to take medications. He was five feet nine inches tall and weighed over 250 pounds.

At the time we had a health assessment tool on the America's Health Network Website. I took Larry through the questions. With a click of the mouse, we had a quantitative answer to the qualitative opinion I had formed, namely, that Larry's life expectancy was dramatically reduced. Worse yet, his quality of life and satisfaction with life stunk. He was unhappy when he called, and he was even more unhappy with my answers.

"Well," he exclaimed, sounding exasperated, "I guess I'll have to go back to the doctor and start taking some pills!"

"Larry," I responded, "pills may help, but until you're willing to partici-pate in your own health care—to take control of your own health—you'll never get better. The pills may slow your decline, but if you truly want to be healthy, you're going to have to develop a strategy to change some things—and change them dramatically and immediately."

He was quiet for a moment. I took a gamble. "Larry, do you have kids?"

I could hear his voice soften. "Yes, two beautiful daughters."

Here was the key I needed. "Do you want to see them be healthy and happy? Graduate from college? Do you want to be there to walk them down the aisle and give them away to their future husbands? Or do you want them to grow up without a dad? Do you want to play with your future grandchildren?"

He was quiet and then almost whispered, "I see what you're saying."

"Then just do what you need to do."

The call ended, and I pretty much forgot about Larry until two years later when, during a commercial break, the producer said, "Walt, we've got an amazing call. It's a guy who says you saved his life." I had no idea who it might be. But, yes, you guessed it—it was Larry.

He didn't sound like the same guy. He described his health journey over the course of the previous two years. He was down to an ideal body weight and was exercising frequently. With his doctor's help, he had changed the diet of his entire family. He found a job he liked more and loved being a dad, now of *three* girls. His blood pressure, blood sugar, and cholesterol levels had nor-malized—initially with medication and then, with his doctor's guidance, going off all his medications through making permanent lifestyle changes. He was excited about how much better he felt.

"Doc, you saved my life."

I smiled and shook my head. "No, Larry. *You* saved your life. And your family will never be the same because of what *you've* done."

I hope I get to meet Larry face-to-face someday. But until then, I tell you this: You can follow this now healthy man's example. So what do you say?

Time to Get Wired

Determine how you will access the Internet, and begin learn-ing how to use it so that you can become more proactive in the way you assess your health. Commit to researching any nonemer-gency health problem you have *before* you make an appointment with your physician. An informed patient is an empowered patient!

HealthCentral.com's LifeView Profile

An excellent place to begin accessing reliable health information on the Internet is HealthCentral.com, the Website of Dr. Dean Edell. Dr. Edell is a well-known medical journalist whose call-in radio program is broadcast across the United States. HealthCentral.com's Website has a number of "Health Profiles" that may be helpful to you (to find these profiles, go to my Website at www.highlyhealthy.net). For these mini-profiles, you'll be asked to answer ten to twenty-five questions and then you'll get personal feedback. As of 2002, mini-profiles were available on

- alcohol and substance abuse,
- sexual health,
- diet and nutrition,
- stress management, and
- exercise and fitness.

HealthCentral's "LifeView" profile gives you a more comprehensive self-evaluation tool. You'll be asked to answer about fifty questions regarding your health. Based on the answers you give, the computer program will estimate your life expectancy and your biggest health risks. The program will tell you your *estimated* health age as compared to your *actual* age, and your life expectancy as compared to your *achievable* life expectancy. You can find this profile at www.highlyhealthy.net.

The program will also review your health risks and tell you which of your risks are below, above, or at the average for the United States population. It will outline your current good health habits and suggest those you might improve or change, tell you the generally recommended preventive health guidelines for your age and gender, and give you follow-up tips selected just for you. You'll also receive helpful links to other Internet sites and newsletters that will give you additional health information.

To get the most out of the LifeView profile, you'll need to know your height and weight; your total cholesterol level, both HDL cholesterol and LDL cholesterol values; and your most recent blood pressure. It's helpful, but not necessary, to also know your body's fat percentage. Your doctor's office can help you gather this information—it's either on your medical chart or can be easily obtained. For any type of health assessment, giving the computer accurate information will give you a more accurate answer. Don't plug in answers you think might be right or better. If you do, you'll only get inaccurate results.

I recently took the LifeView profile, and it informed me that I may be able to add a couple years to my life expectancy by making some simple changes in lifestyle. In my case, my risk for heart attack, stroke, and hypertensive heart disease are all above normal, while my risk for diabetes and lung cancer are below normal.

The program affirmed some things I'm currently doing (or not doing) as "good health habits." For example, I have a healthy blood pressure, don't smoke, always use my seat belt, don't drive under the influence of alcohol or drugs, and don't ride with drivers who are under the influence of alcohol or drugs. I have adequate fiber in my diet and have a healthy total cholesterol level. I have not had work-related injuries in the past year and don't use intravenous drugs or share needles with others.

As for things I could change or do better, the program recommended that I reduce my weight by means of improving my diet and that I consider getting additional exercise. It also recommended that I don't exceed the speed limit while driving, that I reduce my stress at work, and that I reduce the amount of saturated fat in my diet. I was also advised to get my blood pressure checked every one to two years, have my cholesterol tested every five years, get a digital rectal prostate exam every year, and get an eye exam with glaucoma screening and a dental exam every six months. Bottom line, I need to practice more of what I preach! I found this health site and its information to be, in general, both accurate and reliable.

Check Your Oil

Take the LifeView profile on HealthCentral.com—as well as any of the mini-profiles that interest you. Then list all the things you are currently doing (or not doing) that are likely to have an impact on your health. What specifically will you consider changing or improving? And when will you begin?

WebMD.com's Health Risk Appraisal

Another Internet site with a useful health inventory is the WebMD site. You can find their "Health-E-Tools" via my Website at www.highlyhealthy.net. I found this health assessment tool more fun to take than the one at the HealthCentral site—there are a number of fun facts to read beside each question. The results of this assessment look different from the one at Health-Central. A table computes the number of deaths in the next ten years for 10,000 men or women of your age. It will tell your *actual* risk, your *achievable* risk, and the risk of the general population.

Check out your health habits. You may find a number of areas where you can improve your health. These assessments can give you a plumb line against which to compare your current health.

Let me share a warning. Don't gloat, as I was tempted to do, when I learned that I was 37 percent better than average. That's nothing to brag about! Why? Simply because the average American is in such terrible health. What's significant about the WebMD site is that it will give you some idea of how your current health measures up against your achievable health.

The WebMD program also gives a number of suggestions for improving your health. For example, in my case it gave the following suggestions—ones the HealthCentral site didn't mention. The WebMD site had information on

- how I could reduce salt in my diet;
- the controversy about using the blood test for prostate cancer (PSA test) as a screening test for men fifty years of age and older (some medical groups recommend it; others oppose it);
- screening options for early detection of colon cancer;
- immunizations I might consider (although it was perplexing that the site did *not* discuss the influenza vaccine);
- home safety options (including smoke alarms and firearm safety issues); and
- a number of dental health options.

Check Your Transmission Fluid

Take the WebMD Health Risk Appraisal. What is your risk of dying during the next decade from one of the top ten causes of death in the United States? Write down the specific suggestions this Website offers on how you could go about improving your physical health. Plan to take action on at least one of these suggestions during the next week.

With the results of these two health assessments in hand, you should have a pretty good idea of some of the ways you can improve your physical health wheel. While these Internet self-appraisals aren't perfect, they'll give you a good idea of some things you can do—some specific things you can change, just as Larry did—in order to become more highly healthy.

Other Risk Assessment Tools

You may want to check out several risk assessment tools or quizzes for a number of potential health problems. You can get to these tools via my Website at www.highlyhealthy.net:

- Carbohydrates: rate your intake
- Check your cholesterol
- Are you getting enough protein in your diet?
- How sleep-deprived are you?
- Is it really a cold?
- Prostate check for men
- Body mass index
- Ideal body weight
- Smoking cessation quiz
- Allergy quiz

Cancer Risk Appraisal

Hundreds of thousands of Americans are cancer survivors; in most cases the cancer was discovered early and was treated. In addition, according to the American Cancer Society, many types of cancers can be prevented by applying some of the principles found in this book.

For those concerned about cancer (especially if you have a family history of cancer or increased risk factors for cancer—such as a history of smoking), the Harvard Center for Cancer Prevention Website can help you assess your risk for various types of cancer and suggest ways to get regular checkups to detect cancer when the potential for cure is greatest.

Not only will this site's risk calculators tell you your risk for any particular type of cancer, but it will also show you how small changes in your lifestyle, habits, or behavior may decrease or increase your cancer risk. You can find this superb site via www.highlyhealthy.net. You'll be able to determine your risk for twelve of the most common cancers: bladder, breast, cervix, colon, kidney, lung, ovary, pancreas, prostate, skin, stomach, and uterus.

Since my dad was diagnosed with colon cancer just a few years ago at the age of seventy-two, I've been concerned about my personal risk. In fact, I've been *very* concerned about my risk—thinking it would be pretty high. A trip to this Website reduced my worries. The program predicted that my colon cancer risk is actually "much below average." The program suggested that I discuss with my physician the option of taking a single baby-strength aspirin tablet (81 milligrams) four to six times a week (which I've now implemented into my daily regimen).

With this simple change, the program showed me that I would have the lowest risk possible in spite of any genetic component related to my dad's colon cancer. Even so, I still needed a screening colonoscopy when I turned fifty. This calculator not only eased my concerns but also suggested ways I could further lower my risk.

Finding Reliable Health Information on the Internet

I hope this brief discussion gives you insight into the important role the Internet can play in the lives of people who want to remain or to become highly healthy. But before we go on, let me give you some advice. Although the sites I've discussed above are superior, many Web health sites are atrocious in my opinion. Since 1997, the reliability of Internet health information has become the concern of a group called the Internet Healthcare Coalition. This coalition is working to provide clear guidance for evaluating online sources of health information—from product- or disease-related sites developed by regulated manufacturers, to peer-reviewed electronic publications, to patient support and discussion groups. The coalition's goal is to develop well-informed Internet health care consumers, professionals, educators, marketers, and media. I'd strongly urge you to take a look at the coalition's tips on evaluating the reliability of online health information and advice—on the Web via www.highlyhealthy.net.

Although a number of other groups are working on ways to certify health sites on the Internet, there are no certifications I can recommend at present. However, the National Health Information Center has a site that recommends organizations it finds to be both helpful and accurate. You can find this site via www.highlyhealthy.net.

Here's an interesting tidbit: according to the Harris Poll, a polling firm that has been taking the public pulse by surveying millions of people from more than ninety countries over the last forty years, 70 million Americans went online between June 1998 and June 1999 looking for health information.

Take a Day for Yourself

Pick a day within the next three months when you will spend at least a half day studying your results on the health assessment tools in this chapter and contemplating the "Ten Commandments of Preventive Medicine." Plan to journal (or talk to someone) about the results and your feelings about them. Consider making an appointment with your primary care physician to get professional feedback regarding your options for improving your health. Seek immediate medical help if any of your self-assessments are critically high.

CHAPTER FIVE

Practice Acceptance and Letting Go

The Essential of Forgiveness

One of my favorite mentors during my time in medical school was a pediatrician. James Upp, M.D., was a deeply spiritual man and was superbly competent as a physician. I loved the rotation I spent in his office. I enjoyed both watching him work and observing how very much he enjoyed his work and his patients—a joy exceeded only by the joy he received from his relationship with his God and his family. He deeply loved them all.

One fateful evening, his youngest daughter, Diane, was driving down a lonely road. A car approached her, and as it passed, one of the young men in the car tossed a concrete block at her car. The block crashed through the windshield of Diane's car at over ninety miles an hour, instantly snuffing out her precious life.

The boys were apprehended and charged with homicide. While they were in jail, something happened that shocked them, their parents, and our town. Dr. Upp visited the parents of the boys to share in their sorrow and to offer them—face-to-face—his forgiveness. Then he stunned even his closest friends by going to the jail to visit the boys and to let them know that he had forgiven them.

Why would Dr. Upp do such a thing? Would you? Dr. Upp knew in his heart, and then placed into action, his belief that hatred is most harmful to the person who hates. He knew he had to let go of his anger and resentment and blame. Then, and only then, could he heal. By forgiving the boys who had killed his daughter, Dr. Upp was not letting them off the hook. He knew that they would and should face punishment and suffer consequences for their actions. However, after the boys were convicted, he took the witness stand to ask the judge for mercy in the sentencing. He had spent time with these boys. He had seen them weep inconsolably for having taken from him one of his most precious blessings. He had seen their remorse and their sorrow. He trusted that his God would take this tragedy and create good.

Dr. Upp had learned that the one responsible for judging other human beings was *not* him but God. He was willing to trust that all vindication would be God's, not his.

Witnessing Dr. Upp's attitudes and actions forever changed me. He demonstrated one of the keys of being highly healthy. Dr. Upp died recently. I miss him. He loved his son and daughters. He loved life. He loved me. He lived and died a highly healthy person.

While in private practice, I saw anger's effect on a patient named Anne. She was a walking time bomb. The problems recorded on her medical chart were chilling: morbid obesity, depression (probably bipolar), hypertension, high cholesterol, peripheral artery disease, asthma and allergies, sleep disorder, chronic dermatitis, and chronic fatigue. On any checklist of risk factors for early death, Anne ranked near the top. Her only enjoyment in and escape from life was her teaching job. Her only exercise was moving to and from the car. Her diet was a nutritional den of iniquity.

She was frequently in my office and had been in the hospital a number of times. She knew every doctor and nurse there. Anne needed to change her life and her lifestyle, but for some reason she couldn't.

"Dr. Walt," she sighed when I once again suggested she see a Christian psychologist who had just joined our practice, "I've been to counselor after counselor. They're no help at all. Whenever I take one step forward, I just seem to lose control and fall two or three steps back."

"Anne," I said rather sternly, "if you want to become healthy and if you want me to continue to serve you, then you and I need to schedule some time with Gil Hanson, our new psychologist. If he can't help *you*, well, at least maybe he can help *me!*"

She looked surprised. Then she laughed.

"OK, OK. I'll go. But just once."

I agreed—not sure what we might be getting into.

Anne's session with Dr. Hanson began innocently enough. Both Anne and I gave brief summaries of the problems she was having and the problems we had in working together.

Gil began to focus on Anne's past. In what seemed like only a few minutes, she told him about watching her father die on the kitchen floor—in front of her five-year-old eyes. She watched her mother become an alcoholic and then marry a man who abused Anne and her sister for a number of years. She watched her mother get beaten whenever she tried to intervene or protect her daughters. When they arrived home from high school one day, Anne and her sister found their mom hanging from an electric cord in the garage—death by suicide.

I was stunned as we watched Anne dissolve into waves of uncontrollable sobbing.

"I didn't know," I muttered to Dr. Hanson. "She never told me any of this."

Gil reached over and squeezed my forearm. "Walt, she couldn't tell anyone until she was ready."

Several years later, after a great deal of work, an increasingly healthier Anne told me, "The anger from my past was eating me alive. If we hadn't dealt with it the way we did, it would've killed me!"

I believe she was right. So how *did* she deal with it? She learned the essential of forgiveness and applied it to her life. The result? I saw her health improve dramatically.

Researchers in San Diego, California, published a survey of more than 20,000 adults, which showed that those who suffered physical, psychological, or emotional abuse as children (or were raised in homes where they experienced or observed physical violence, substance abuse, mental illness, or criminal behavior) were far more likely, as adults, to develop serious illnesses—such as heart disease, asthma, bronchitis, diabetes, and cancer. These researchers surmise that hostile experiences in childhood underlie the most common causes of death in America. The cause points to the anger, anxiety, and depression produced in the young victims of these terrible experiences. When these kids are growing up, they often self-medicate their pain with behaviors such as overeating, smoking, and using drugs or alcohol—which they often find to be effective coping devices tending to lead to chronic use. Clearly, then, these early traumatic experiences can be a huge roadblock to becoming a highly healthy person.

Many other researchers have concluded that there are a multitude of ways that the unresolved trauma, shock, or ordeals of one's childhood can stand in the way of high degrees of health. There are dozens of studies demonstrating that the chronic stress caused by unresolved emotional pain causes damage to the immune system and the circulatory system. What's more, it can also depress vital cardiac function, hormone levels, and other physical functions.

For anyone who has suffered as a result of another's actions—and that includes every last one of us—I have this prescription: *We must make peace with our past.* We must undertake the daunting task of learning to accept what we cannot change and let go of our pain and anger over the ways we have been hurt. Our lives may literally depend on it.

Forgiveness Starts with You

Find a comfortable place to sit and relax. Be sure to have your journal and a pen with you. Close your eyes for a moment, thinking about this question: Is there someone who has hurt, harmed, wounded, or damaged me—even unknowingly?

As you think about this person and this hurt, notice what your body does. Does it tense up? Do you feel flushed or angry? Is your pulse starting to race? Are you trembling or breathing quickly? Do you feel pain?

This is unpleasant, isn't it?

Begin to ponder how these feelings are harming your health. Imagine the damage these thoughts are doing to your heart and blood vessels and soul. Wouldn't it be in your best interest to let these destructive feelings go?

As an act of your will, practice thinking about the person and the harmful situation, and then whisper out loud, "_____, I forgive you."

Let out a slow deep breath. Imagine blowing out all your anger. Yes, your anger may be justified, but it also could be killing you. Blow it out.

I realize that practicing forgiveness for deep hurts is a complex and difficult act. I can assure you that you will begin to experience positive results as you learn how to *practice* letting go of your pain.

F-O-R-G-I-V-I-N-G

Countless books have been written on the subject of forgiveness, acceptance, and letting go of situations and people we cannot control. The resources you have to draw on to help you find emotional freedom and serenity are plentiful. For my patients, I've offered the following prescription—based on the acrostic F-O-R-G-I-V-I-N-G—to help them with the difficult and emotionally painful task of healing from past hurts.

F = Forgiving Is Highly Healthy

When people are hurt, they almost instinctively try to protect themselves or hide the hurt. Sometimes they even deny the hurt. Sometimes, though rarely, they will consciously "forget" the hurt. It's almost as though they believe that if they don't think about, talk about, or deal with the hurt, it won't bother them. But this just isn't true. Harboring anger or hurt or resentment always gnaws away like a cancer at a person's happiness and health.

If you have not forgiven someone, then for *your* sake (not necessarily for the sake of the person who hurt you) consider forgiving him or her. This requires some difficult and potentially painful steps. It will require you to remember and relive the pain. For my patients who have wrestled with for-giveness, I've prescribed that they actually start with an empty journal and just begin writing. I want them to recall the event as objectively as possible— almost as an observer.

I encourage them not to waste their time venting hatred or ill feelings against the person or persons who caused the pain—nor should they waste their time wishing for an apology. I especially encourage them not to dwell on their role as a victim. I want them to recognize that a wrong was indeed com-mitted—and then to clearly describe and illustrate that wrong, objectively, in writing. This is the first, and maybe most important, step in forgiving.

I've found that my patients who wrestle with a painful past can benefit greatly by attempting to find as much value as possible in their past affliction or disaster. By actively looking for the good that came from your suffering, you'll be much more likely to both counterbalance and then negate its harm-ful effects. We don't have the power to change the past, but we do have a great deal of control over how we experience the past *now.*

The Nazi concentration camps of World War II led to the destruction of millions of lives—but not all of those who "died" were physically killed. Many continue, even today, to be destroyed by the experiences they had in those brutal prisons. They are still prisoners of their past.

However, there are Holocaust survivors who, in spite of their indescribably horrible experiences, have allowed their pain to be turned into good. For exam-ple, Auschwitz survivors Corrie ten Boom and Diet Eman have written and spo-ken extensively about how they had a choice: They could continue to respond in the habitual way when painful past events came to mind, namely continuing to hate their tormentors, or they could look at what God had accomplished in them through the terror. When they began to do this, they could focus on the positive things that came to them from these events. They were able to see that their past actually made them stronger, refined them more purely, and gave them life lessons they could use to strengthen and equip others. Although Corrie is now deceased, her writings still make an impact around the world.

When I had the privilege of meeting Diet Eman, I asked her, "What would have become of you had you given in to the hatred and bitterness of your pain and loss?"

She took a deep breath. Her bright eyes looked away, as though gazing down a long tunnel to her past. She furrowed her heavily wrinkled brow. "Dr. Larimore, it would have killed me. But instead it gives me life."

One final thought here: I find some patients who, when reliving the pain, find themselves wrestling with a great deal of shame—particularly those who are victims of sexual exploitation and abuse.

I've told my patients that I consider shame to be a cancer of the spirit. Shame has so many negative effects. If you are living with shame, then it will be virtually impossible for you to become a highly healthy person. Shame makes you feel worthless, undeserving, and unlovable. Shame is different from guilt or remorse. Feeling guilty (or remorseful) is feeling bad about things *you have done* (or failed to do) in the past. Shame is feeling bad about *who you are.*

The surest way to overcome this form of shame is to begin to understand who you are from God's point of view (see chapter 9). Without banishing shame from your soul, the rest of this process will not continue. If you are not able to do this, I encourage you to seek professional pastoral counseling.

Finding the Good in the Bad

Find a quiet place and think about the situations and people that have populated your past. On a piece of paper, list on one side all of the horrible things about your past. Then on the other side, list all of the positive characteristics these events created in you— list all of the good that came in spite of the bad.

This will *not* be an easy exercise—in and of itself it may be very painful. But the positives that come from this exercise can be lifelong.

O = Organize Your Thoughts by Writing

Writing, especially journaling, is a powerful tool for recognizing and releasing pain. You can use it to enrich your health.

David Hager, M.D., a professor, an obstetrician-gynecologist, and my close friend, has developed a method for releasing the pain of losing a child. In his practice, he cares for many women who have lost children to miscarriages or to abortions performed by others. He offers a ceremony for these women and their husbands in which the mom or the couple is invited to bury a letter that she or they have written to their lost child. Dr. Hager describes the experience as overwhelmingly emotional, but one that leads to healing.

In the same way, I've recommended that my patients who struggle with unreleased past pain use the powerful healing tool of writing—even if they don't consider themselves to be writers. One prescription I've given is to have my patients write a letter to the one(s) who hurt them. I encourage my patients not to judge or censor their writing, not to hold back any emotion, not to worry about grammar. Just let it all come out. I suggest they keep this letter private. It is not a letter to send to the person who hurt them but to use as a tool for personal healing—and then to destroy.

A former patient back in rural North Carolina, a soldier unable to let go of the pain of the Vietnam War, took me up on this advice. I still remember a phone call from him at 2:00 A.M.

"Walt," he almost shouted, "you won't believe it. It's gone!"

"Who is this? What are you talking about?" I asked, being roused from a deep sleep.

"Walt, this is Tim Johnson. I did it. I did it. It worked. It really worked."

"Tim, you did what?"

"Walt, I wrote the letters. I wrote Sarge and Binky. I wrote the Cong. I even wrote Johnson and Nixon. I tell you, I was one angry guy. But, Walt, it's gone. It's gone!"

He broke into sobs for what seemed like several minutes. As he composed himself, I asked, "Tim, are you OK, buddy?"

"Walt, I've never been better. The pain's gone. I feel so much better. I want to bury these guys. Will you come over and help me?"

"You bet, Tim. I'll be right there."

I rolled out of bed. Barb didn't move. Over the years, she had grown used to me leaving during the night to attend a hospital admission or a birth.

The evening air was cool. Tim's house was just a few miles away, nestled in a small hollow. When I drove up, he met me on the front porch.

"Follow me," he instructed.

We walked to the edge of the backyard. He had dug a hole, and I could see the shovel and a pile of dirt in the moonlight. He pulled a roll of papers from his belt, knelt down, and gently placed them in the bottom of the hole. He struck a match, and we watched his hatred burn to ash.

"Doc, I know you're a man of prayer. Would you say one for me—and Sarge—and Binky?"

So I prayed. Then together we filled that hole with dirt. We buried that pain. It was gone. And so are a bunch of Tim's diseases. That day he took a huge step on the path toward a higher degree of health.

Bury Your Pain

Is there even a shred of shame or pain haunting your soul? Spend some time thinking through your life. Jot down any item of shame or pain on the last page of your journal.

Plan a date with a person who loves you deeply and whom you trust implicitly. If you don't have someone, consider doing this exercise with a pastoral professional. At this get-together, share these items with your friend or counselor. Until you can discuss these types of things with someone else, you will neither be free of them nor highly healthy.

After you've completely discussed these issues, tear out the piece of paper—in the presence of your friend—and either bury it or burn it. Afterward, thank God for being big enough to handle all your pain and all your shame. Let it go.

R = Review Your Experience

This step has two parts. The first requires you to review what you experienced, but this time you'll do it through the eyes of the person(s) who hurt you. In the second part, you'll need to remember the forgiveness you've been given by others. Some of my patients have found that this task takes the most time in thought, meditation, and prayer, for in this step I ask them to practice a little-used skill: *empathy.* I tell my patients that empathy is the ability to see things from another person's perspective or point of view. Empathy involves an effort to feel that person's feelings, seeking to figure out and understand his or her motivations and identify with the pressures that may have driven that person to hurt them or cause them pain. This can be difficult indeed.

But what if you come up empty? What if you can't begin to imagine why someone would do what was done to you—and you can't find anyone who can explain it to you? Dale's solution might work for you.

For decades, Dale had lived with the pain caused by his high school football coach. Dale wasn't much of an athlete, but he tried out for and made his high school team. He was delighted to be part of the "in crowd." He didn't play much, but he was on the squad. As it turned out, he played in just enough of each game to qualify for a varsity letter. He had dreamed of "lettering" in a varsity sport since he was a little boy. He pictured himself wearing his letter jacket. He delighted in the approving looks he would get.

However, at the end of the season, Coach Keaton called him into the office. "Dale, I've changed the qualifications for lettering. I've raised the number of required quarters, and you don't qualify. I'm sorry, son. This is my first year as coach. I need to do this. I want to set a precedent that will help the team."

Dale left the office without a word. He was crushed. When I met him, nearly thirty years later, he was still living with the anger and resentment he had toward Coach Keaton—although I didn't know that when he first came to see me. His chief complaint was fatigue and trouble sleeping. It took time to get to the heart of the issue—but when I did, I explained the F-O-R-G-I-V-I-N-G process to Dale, and he agreed to give it a try. The "F" and "O" steps weren't easy for him—dredging up a lot of uncomfortable feelings he'd been suppressing for nearly thirty years. The third step—to see things from the coach's perspective— was nearly impossible. He couldn't begin to imagine why Coach Keaton had done that. He even talked to our town's football coach, who could offer no reasonable explanation. We were at an impasse. What could I suggest to Dale?

Thankfully, I didn't have to suggest anything. Dale came up with a brilliant idea all by himself. He decided to write a letter to himself as though he were Coach Keaton. In the letter, Dale—writing as the coach—tried to explain the harmful act. It was a difficult step for Dale, which took a fair amount of time, thought, and prayer. But he did it.

The results were amazing. Almost immediately Dale began to sense that he was being set free from his decades-long hatred and resentment. While he didn't agree with the coach's decision, he was ready to proceed to the point of forgiveness and letting go of his pain.

My friend James had lost his leg in a North Vietnamese booby trap during the Vietnam War. His hatred for Vietnamese people was intense—and it was eroding his health. He suffered from anxiety, depression, chest pain, and high blood pressure. Yet he suffered most from the weight of his hatred.

One day he accepted my challenge to begin practicing F-O-R-G-I-V-I-N-G. Like Dale, the third step of seeking to understand what happened from the viewpoint of those who hurt him was his most difficult. I saw him several months later. He reported that all of his symptoms were gone. With a doctor's supervision, he was able to wean off all of his medications. "Doc, I'm sleeping like a baby!" he declared. His blood pressure and pulse were normal. He looked like a new man.

"What did you do, James?"

"Well, I wrote those letters. First, I pretended I was Charlie. So I wrote a letter from Charlie to me. I wrote how I hated him—for invading my country—for raping and killing my people. It took a long time, Doc. I had to do a lot of reading about the Vietnamese. Even talked to one of their army veterans I met here in town."

He paused for a moment.

"Then," he continued slowly, as though telling the story about someone else, "James wrote Charlie back." Tears were beginning to well up in James's eyes. "It was the hardest letter James ever wrote. Took him days. He had a lot of questions for Charlie. But he wrote it and Charlie wrote him back." Now tears were streaming down James's face.

"I heard about a medical mission going to Vietnam. I signed up. Just got back last month. I met a hundred Charlies. I ministered to them. But, more important, they ministered to me."

The pain was still very real. James still faces life without one of his legs. But he was no longer carrying his heavy load. James chose, as an act of *his* will, to take this crucial step on the road to becoming more highly healthy.

James's and Dale's work to develop the skill of empathy prepared them for the next part in the process of reviewing their experience—to recall the gifts of forgiveness that others had given to them. In this step, I instructed each of them to make a list of all the things for which others had forgiven them—beginning with their parents.

Think how many times you received forgiveness from your parents. How many times has your spouse or a sibling forgiven you for something? Have you ever harmed or offended or wounded someone who later forgave you? As you think back on these events, recall how you felt when you caused harm. Think of the guilt you felt. Then remember how you felt when you were forgiven.

Most of my patients tell me they felt free when they were given the gift of forgiveness—as though the chains were broken. By recalling and journaling about as many episodes as possible in which you were forgiven, and then remembering and journaling about how it felt to be forgiven, it's likely that you'll develop the desire to give this gift of freedom to people who have hurt you.

People who understand and deeply appreciate that they have been forgiven by God and others are usually profoundly grateful for their emotional freedom—and forgiven people are usually motivated to extend the forgiveness they have received.

G = Give the Boot to Anger and Regret

Anger

The young man was especially pleased. He served on a prestigious teen advisory board for one of the most respected clothing stores in his hometown. His grandmother, whom he loved and admired, had come for a visit.

He was looking forward to taking both his mother and grandmother to his store, where he was known and liked. In fact, because of his advisory board position, he was treated like a very important person. With his somewhat low self-esteem, the young man's visits to the store were like a cup of cold water to a nomad in a scorching desert.

One of the perks of being on the advisory board was having a specially marked parking place at the front of the store—a perk he was sure would impress his grandmother.

His mother was driving that day. As she pulled up to the store, her son was thrilled to see that the special parking place was open. (You see, others were allowed to park there as well.) As his mom drove toward the favored spot, his pride began to swell. He knew how proud his mom and grandmother would be—it was his day to shine!

Then, to his horror, a car sped into the parking lot, turned in front of their car, and pulled into *his* parking place.

Something inside him exploded. He jumped from his mother's car and ran to the intruder's car. He ripped open the door and unleashed a crimson-faced verbal barrage that flooded the entire parking lot.

The recipient of this fusillade was shocked speechless. Never had she been so berated. She frequently parked in the spot. Her husband owned the store. She apologized profusely—which seemed to stem the vociferous torrent of abuse—then pulled out to park in another spot. The young man then directed his dumbfounded mother and grandmother into *his* parking place.

Do you think this young man might grow up to become an angry, easily irritated, abrupt, intolerant, and harsh kind of person? Would you be comfortable being around such a person? Can't you see him growing up with no real friends, and certainly no admirers? Can't you see him dying of a heart attack at the age of forty-five?

Well, in fact, he's at risk for exactly such an outcome. Anger is lethal.

In their best-selling book *Anger Kills,* authors Redford and Virginia Williams point to dozens of studies that show that anger is not just another negative emotion but something that can kill. Anger can lead to heart disease, heart attacks, heart rhythm irregularities, and many other life-threatening diseases. The authors point out that a person who fails to recognize and deal with his or her anger is just like someone who each day takes a small dose of a poison. Eventually, it makes the entire system toxic and can literally lead to death.

I'm not talking about people who get appropriately angry from time to time. In fact, the Bible tells us, "In your anger do not sin." Occasional anger that is justified but temporary—for example, when you are treated unfairly—is not wrong or harmful. However, when anger is a constant companion—one you can't leave behind—then your anger will prevent you from becoming a highly healthy person.

Check Your Hostility Dipstick

Are you at risk to experience the unhealthy side effects of being habitually angry? Take The Relationships Questionnaire in appendix 1. This remarkable questionnaire will help you determine your *hostility index*—the degree to which the "anger toxin" is in your system. Highly healthy people are those who, by nature and design, are not hostile—or have learned to set their anger aside.

If your hostility index is low, that's great news. If it isn't, then read on and follow the subsequent prescriptions.

Regret

Although not as pernicious as anger, regret can also rob us of our health. "If only I hadn't . . ." or "I wish I had . . ." or "I should have . . ."—these statements of regret do nothing but cause more pain. One of the most important aspects of finding healing for old pain and of overcoming past mistakes is to stop punishing yourself. You have to develop a strategy to forgive yourself and resolve to think and act differently toward yourself. You cannot be highly healthy if the rot of regret lives in your heart.

Do you carry a shameful regret? Review your regrets, clarify who you were at the time, what you knew and didn't know, what choices you were aware of at the time. Is the choice you made—under those circumstances—most likely the one you would make again, given those same circumstances?

Or perhaps you've clearly made a mistake—or a series of mistakes. Then you have an opportunity before you. You can use the poor choices of the past to grow and to become more mature *now*. God is willing to forgive you. The Bible teaches, "If we claim to be without sin [that we've never wronged others], we deceive ourselves and the truth is not in us. If we confess [admit] our sins, [God] is faithful and just and will forgive us our sins and purify us from all unrighteousness. If we claim we have not sinned, we make him out to be a liar and his word has no place in our lives."

Our job is to admit that we've been wrong to foster our anger, bitterness, shame, or regrets. Admitting that we were wrong to hold on to these emotions is a form of confession. And in the Bible, to *confess* is simply to agree with God that the attitudes or emotions or actions we've had or done are wrong. We can begin to find healing when we simply agree that we missed the mark, that we fell short.

Making our confession to God and seeking his forgiveness does not preclude our responsibility to admit our wrongdoing to those we've harmed and to ask for their forgiveness as well. Nor does it absolve us of our responsibility to make restitution whenever possible. Nevertheless, medical science confirms that confession and forgiveness have strong healing benefits.

Knowing that the Creator of the universe, who designed each of us, is willing and able to completely forgive all of our past wrongs allows us to begin the process of forgiving ourselves—and to ask others to forgive us as well.

Confession Is Good for Health

If there are things in your past that you regret—wrongs you've done and not yet dealt with—list them in your journal.

First, pray about these issues. If you need to confess any wrong to God, do so—knowing that with this confession come forgiveness and cleansing. Afterward, thank God that he has forgiven your wrongdoing. Bill Bright calls this *spiritual breathing.* You exhale (confess) the bad, and then inhale the good (the forgiveness and filling of God).

Second, if there are people you have wronged who are still alive, consider visiting them or calling them to admit your wrongdoing and to ask for their forgiveness. Even if they refuse to forgive you, your decision to seek forgiveness will assist in your healing.

Third, if you've never forgiven those who have wronged you, consider visiting or calling them to confess the anger or bitterness that has been in your heart. Then forgive them and tell them that you've forgiven them. They may choose not to receive the forgiveness, but your giving it, sincerely and with a pure heart, will increase your health and will set you free.

I = Invest in Removing Resentment

Thinking negatively about yourself is certainly unhealthy, but holding a grudge or harboring anger against others is also harmful to your health. King Solomon wrote about the way in which unresolved resentments alienate friends: "He who covers over an offense promotes love, but whoever repeats the matter separates close friends."

The Bible says that if we've done nothing to mend fractured relationships with the people God has put in our lives, worshiping and trying to please God aren't going to pass muster. This holds true for any significant relationship in which a soul-damaging wound has occurred. Even if the fault is with the other person, it is *our* responsibility to seek healing in the relationship. Jesus taught, "If you are offering your gift at the altar and there remember that your brother has something against you, leave your gift there in front of the altar. First go and be reconciled to your brother; then come and offer your gift."

Of course, there are times when reconciliation seems impossible. You may be in such a situation with a friend or family member right now. In cases like these, continue to pray for the people from whom you're estranged, dress the wounds as much as possible, and then leave the rest to God. Nothing preserves and even increases the unhealthy power of past pain more than rehashing the events over and over. Perpetually lamenting and grieving over your past will not only *not* help you find healing, it may well cause disease that will prevent you from being healthy. It's like watching the same horror movie again and again, while praying that the way the movie ends would change. Instead, you must learn to turn off the movie, leave the theater, and move on with your life.

The inner peace that increases your odds of being a highly healthy person comes from accepting your past and then moving out with hope and confidence into your future. By beginning to accept your past as something your Creator can use to improve your future—to improve who and what you are—you can then concentrate on seeing what he is doing, what he is accomplishing in and through your life. You can blame him, curse him, and ceaselessly ask, "Why me, God? Why did you let this happen to me?" Or you can *choose* to accept what he has allowed and begin to seek the answer to much more profitable questions: "God, what are you trying to teach me? What are you doing here?" These questions attest to a childlike trust in God's goodness, wisdom, and plan. As you begin to seek the good that can result even from bad things, you can see his hand at work in all things.

Highly healthy people simply are not blamers—they can't be. The more you blame yourself or resent others for your painful past, the more harm you do to your own health. Highly healthy people take responsibility for their thoughts and actions. They are willing to wrestle with their own shame, guilt, and anger—and to subdue it.

Take responsibility for your feelings. Fix whatever is wrong if you can. Apologize. Accept punishment. Make restitution. Admit your wrongdoing to God and ask for forgiveness. And don't do it again. Choose to banish grudges and resentments—to let them go so you can be set free. Make the *conscious choice* to forgive—even if you have to practice forgiveness over and over.

V = Victory Comes in Forgiving Others

A study conducted at the University of Michigan's Institute of Social Research affirmed what previous studies had already discovered: People who forgive themselves and others are less likely to suffer from various forms of psychological distress such as nervousness, restlessness, and hopelessness.

Dr. Loren L. Toussaint, who carried out the research at the University of Michigan, reported that a lot of us are endangering our health by holding on to guilt and resentment. This national survey revealed that 75 percent of the adult participants claimed that they believed God had forgiven them for their own past transgressions. However, only 52 percent reported that they had forgiven others, and not even half of those surveyed had forgiven themselves for harming others.

So if you're one of the many folks who believe the old adage, "To err is human, to forgive divine," take note that medical science is proving that "to forgive is healthy." Without learning the habit of forgiveness, you cannot be a highly healthy person.

The next step, then, is a step of commitment. Make a lifelong promise—a covenant—to forgive those who hurt you. You must understand, though, that it is impossible to "forgive and forget." In nearly every case, you won't be able to literally forget what happened. Don't even try. Forgiveness is not forgetting; rather, it is determining to treat the person who harmed you as though the hurt never happened. It is a decision—an act of the will—to treat the person as though he or she had never done the harm.

I've had patients struggle mightily with this step. After they make the decision to forgive but then find themselves remembering the event or the pain, they often think this is proof that they must not have truly forgiven. They have believed a lie, namely, that to really forgive someone, you must forgive *and* forget.

This step can take many forms—telling someone you've forgiven the person who hurt you, writing or calling the one who harmed you to let him know that you've forgiven him. But the one step I suggest to all my patients at this point in the process is that they fill out a *certificate of forgiveness.* On the certificate they write that they have, as of that day, chosen to forgive. They then sign and date the certificate and place it in their journal.

It's worth repeating one more time: Forgiving someone for something she's done against you or to you does *not* condone or sanction her behavior. It does not excuse her from her actions or even the consequences of her wrongs. It doesn't mean that you can't be cautious when interacting with this person. However, forgiving others, even if they are ignorant of what they have done, is a necessary part of *your* becoming highly healthy. Do you remember the words of Jesus on the cross? "Father, forgive them, for they do not know what they are doing."

Give Out "I Forgive You" Awards

Almost all word-processing programs have certificates you can adapt and print. If you can't find one, create one on a piece of paper. Put CERTIFICATE OF FORGIVENESS as the title. On the certificate, write the names of those whom you have chosen to forgive as of today. Then sign and date the certificate and keep it as a visual reminder of the decision you've made.

I've had some patients who at this point have come to realize that their primary anger or feeling of resentment is aimed at God—not at the person who actually harmed them. Do you ever wonder, *How could a loving God allow . . . ?* or, *If God* really *loved me, then why . . . ?* If this describes you, consider the potential health benefits of filling out a certificate of forgiveness for God—then signing and dating it.

Let me be abundantly clear: God does not need your forgiveness. He is just and perfect. Yet *you* may need to work through this exercise, coming to the point where you consciously ask God to forgive you for blaming him, admitting that your bitterness toward him was unfounded and misplaced. If you're willing to do that, now is the time. Fill out the certificate and then, in prayer, admit your wrong and then immediately accept his love and forgiveness. Although this can be a difficult exercise, it is necessary if you've harbored bitterness toward God and if you want to be a highly healthy person.

Making forgiveness a habit takes practice. In my experience, the emotional and spiritual healing that comes from forgiveness can only begin after someone makes a decision to forgive and follows through with that decision. However, forgiveness is also a *process* that may take a long time. This is especially true if the physical, emotional, spiritual, or relational wounds are severe. Continuing to experience the memories of your pain is *not* proof that your hard work of forgiveness is for naught. It merely proves that you haven't forgotten what happened, and that's OK.

Once the healing process begins, you'll notice that your emotional orientation toward the person who hurt you will begin to change. This is a remarkable process. Researchers tell us that these changes will actually filter not only into your beliefs and behaviors but also into your body and brain biochemistry.

Even your facial expressions, posture, and body language will change. Both your blood pressure and heart function are likely to improve. Bottom line: Forgiveness heals both the person who is forgiven and the person who forgives.

I = Increase Your Gratitude for Past Pain

Once you've come this far in the F-O-R-G-I-V-I-N-G journey, you may begin to notice a strange sensation—a faint sense of gratitude for your past pain. Maybe you've begun to see how your mistakes—or how others have wronged you—have resulted in positive changes in your character. Maybe you've begun to see the seedlings of *good* beginning to grow out of the ashes of hurt and the ruins of burned-out dreams.

When Barb and I were studying in Europe, we made a trek into Morocco. In the old city of Fez, we were taken to a gold smelter. In the unbelievably hot building, craftsmen were refining gold ore into pure gold. Chunks of ore were placed into small cauldrons and heat was applied with a propane blowtorch. As the ore began to melt, the smelter would ladle off the dross that rose to the surface and then turn up the heat. Our guide told us that if the heat was applied too quickly or for too long, the gold would be ruined.

Noticing that no thermometers were being used, I asked the guide how the smelter could tell when there had been enough heat applied. Our guide replied, "The gold will be pure when the craftsman sees his reflection in the gold."

The implication of this simple statement rocked my soul. Barb and I talked throughout supper and into the evening. Could it be that the pain in our lives was a form of heat, allowed or applied by our Creator to refine us— to allow others to see his reflection in our lives? Now, nearly twenty-five years later, I've come to believe that this is exactly the process that God allows to occur in our lives.

Only after we can begin to accept—and maybe even welcome—the pain from the past, only when we can begin to feel a twinge of rejoicing in the suffering we've experienced, can we move to the next step, namely, cultivating gratitude for past pain.

No matter what happened in the past, no matter how horrible your memories, try to look for all the gifts for which you can be thankful. You may be shocked to find that you can even become grateful for your past pain *just because* of what you learned from it and the ways in which your character has been fueled and refined by it.

Is this beginning to make sense ? Does it help you begin to understand the seemingly strange teaching of the Bible when it says, "Dear friends, do not be surprised at the painful trial you are suffering, as though something strange were happening to you. But rejoice . . ."? Or, "We also rejoice in our sufferings, because we know that suffering produces perseverance; perseverance, character; and character, hope. And hope does not disappoint us . . ."

One prescription I've written to patients wrestling with emotional pain is to pray the Old Testament psalms. If you don't have a copy, many bookstores sell a collection of the psalms in easy-to-understand language. I've found in my own life—and it's been true for many of my patients as well—that using the psalms to pray to God can be instructive and profoundly helpful. The psalmists knew pain and regret, guilt and remorse. Their prayers can become our own.

For the person who has a personal relationship with God and who is growing spiritually, it is indeed possible—in fact, probable—that gratitude, even for suffering, will slowly but surely develop. In writing to the Colossians, the apostle Paul taught this very principle: "So then, just as you received Christ Jesus as Lord, continue to live in him, rooted and built up in him, strengthened in the faith as you were taught, and overflowing with thankfulness." Highly healthy people become thankful people—full of a gratitude that overflows—even in the midst of pain and suffering.

N = Navigate to Inner Peace

No matter how much trauma my patients have experienced, I've found that, as they apply the F-O-R-G-I-V-I-N-G process, they can begin to find healing and inner peace. This peace is based on peace with others, peace with self, and, most important, peace with God.

Many people try to find inner peace through treatments or therapies such as meditation, yoga, aromatherapy, massage, a hot bath, calming music, a walk in a peaceful setting, deep breathing, focusing on pleasant memories, self-hypnosis, and a host of other things. While each of these may bring a transient calm in the midst of life's many storms, none of these are a source of permanent peace—inner peace.

I believe that no person can have a true and lasting inner peace until he or she has found peace with their Creator—their God. Only then can he or she have a peace that "transcends all understanding." This ancient Scripture that is as alive as today's news says, "Let your gentleness be evident to all. The Lord is near. Do not be anxious about anything, but in everything, by prayer and petition, with thanksgiving, present your requests to God. And the peace of God, which transcends all understanding, will guard your hearts and your minds."

Sounds like a highly healthy person, wouldn't you agree? In chapter 8 I'll spend more time discussing this principle.

G = Give Comfort to Others

The final phase of the F-O-R-G-I-V-I-N-G process involves using the healing that comes from forgiveness to reach out to others—to comfort them in their pain. The Scriptures teach that God "comforts us in all our troubles, so that we can comfort those in any trouble with the comfort we ourselves have received from God." Part of finding healing from past pain and mistakes—part of becoming a highly healthy person—is sharing our pain and our healing process with others who are not as far down the path as we are.

After the births of our daughter, Kate, and our son, Scott, Barb and I lost four children to miscarriage in the third or fourth month of pregnancy. The pain was unimaginable. I was shocked to find that each loss was emotionally more difficult than the one before. After each miscarriage, we couldn't look at another couple's baby without having feelings of jealousy and contempt. We were angry with God and with each other.

Our road to healing was long, and it involved many of the same steps I've recommended to you. I've practiced what I'm preaching here. It works. We finally came to peace with our losses through using the steps I've outlined. We could begin to see the good that God accomplished in us and through us, individually and as a couple, as a result of these terrible events. Gradually we began to receive comfort—and even peace.

But for us, a profoundly healing step was taken when we began to minister to other couples who were experiencing the heartbreak of their own miscarriage. Comforting others with the comfort with which we had been comforted truly resulted in more comfort. By giving comfort, we received it.

DISPENSING MERCY AND GRACE

There you have it. To become a highly healthy person, you must practice acceptance and letting go. You must practice forgiving. In his famous 1828 dictionary, Noah Webster defined forgiving as "pardoning; remitting; inclined to overlook offenses; mild; merciful; compassionate."

Justice is giving to others what they deserve. Mercy is not giving what is deserved. Grace is giving what is not deserved. Highly healthy people are liberal in mercy and grace. Are you? If not, spend some time reading and then applying the message of the third essential of highly healthy people.

CHAPTER SIX

Lighten Your Load

The Essential of Reducing SADness (Stress, Anxiety, and Depression)

The impact of the terrorist attacks of September 11, 2001, on the health of Americans has reverberated across our country long past that dreadful day. Although feelings of national pride and patriotism soared in the months after 9/11, personal attitudes turned from generally positive to alarmingly negative. By the end of 2001, doctors were beginning to see a dramatic increase in the number of patients with insomnia, nightmares, stomachaches, irritability, and an inability to concentrate.

Dr. Mark Schuster, a researcher with the Rand Corporation, found that many people reacted to the 9/11 attacks as though they had been attacked personally. Feelings of loss of well-being were felt across all age groups and all sections of the country. Even people who lived in places where there were no tall buildings or military facilities experienced substantial stress levels.

The Rand researchers found that about 44 percent of the adults surveyed reported one or more substantial symptoms of stress. At least 90 percent of those responding to the Rand researchers admitted experiencing at least low levels of potentially unhealthy stress symptoms.

Interestingly, Americans responded to this incredible national affront to their emotional health by seeking closer ties to family. Scores turned from picking up meals at fast-food pickup windows to dining with family and friends. Many began walking or taking up other forms of exercise. Others plugged into a wide variety of social support systems—including church, synagogue, and support group attendance. Many turned to religion for spiritual support. Many gave away their time and their money. Virtually everyone checked on the safety of his or her loved ones. Most watched or took part in memorial vigils held around the nation. In short, the citizens of the United States illustrated the importance of combating anxiety, depression, and stress with positive action. Let's look briefly at how this principle can dramatically improve your health.

A positive outlook on life has been shown to improve the quality of life and prolong its length. Over the last decade, research provided solid evidence that "looking on the bright side" can both prevent heart disease and minimize its consequences in those who have it.

For example, researchers from Johns Hopkins University found that those with optimistic personalities were only half as likely as their more pessimistic counterparts to experience a heart event. In other words, positive attitudes seemed to protect these folks from serious illness and death. The findings support the results of previous research linking pessimism with higher levels of anger, anxiety, and depression—emotions that may be risk factors for heart disease.

Researchers in Canada reviewed sixteen studies (spanning thirty years) that examined patients' attitudes toward health—particularly attitudes after surgery. "In each case," said Donald Cole of the Institute for Work and Health in Toronto, "the better a patient's expectations about how they would do after surgery or some health procedure, the better they did." However, participants who suffered from depression (and a negative outlook toward their disease)—a flattened emotional wheel—were dramatically less likely to stick to a healthy lifestyle to keep their physical, spiritual, and relational wheels lubricated, inflated, and balanced.

The Johns Hopkins study and multiple other studies are reaching this conclusion: A healthy mind and positive attitude can lead to a healthier mind and a healthier body.

Can a positive attitude help you become a more highly healthy person? By all means—especially to the extent that it helps reduce heart disease, the biggest killer of Americans, both male and female. In fact, many female callers to my radio show seem stunned to learn that their risk of dying from cardiovascular disease (heart attack, heart disease, vascular disease, or stroke) is seven to ten times higher than their risk of dying from all forms of cancer combined (see chapter 4 for more details).

ASSESSING YOUR EMOTIONAL HEALTH WHEEL

Here are some ways to assess your emotional health wheel. Among the most common emotional problems that prevent people from becoming highly healthy are stress, anxiety, and depression.

Evaluating Stress

Plain old *stress* is very likely the most common problem that can weaken the emotional wheel of health. Stress is virtually unavoidable in contemporary life. In one national survey, over 90 percent of Americans reported high levels of stress at least several times a week. I can't tell you how many of my patients have told me that they feel like they are running about as fast as they can. Nearly all of them report that they feel stressed.

For the purposes of this book I'll define *stress* as "any change that requires you to adapt or change the way you are doing something." Stress can come from big things—retirement, a job change, a pregnancy, a new baby, moving, the loss of a loved one, attending a new school, or beginning a new job. Stress can also come from little things—a surprise schedule change, a change in the weather, a flat tire or traffic jam, a sudden deadline, misplaced house keys, or an electrical outage. Technically, physicians call these events *stressors*. But I'll use the words *stress* and *stressors* to mean the same thing.

Some stress is good. In fact, we are designed, I believe, to act in response to certain amounts of stress. It can help us grow—physically, emotionally, relationally, and spiritually. In the physical realm, our body is in constant flux. For example, our bones are constantly being dissolved and new bone being laid down. With the right amount of stress, our bones become thicker and stronger. In the mental and emotional realm, certain amounts of stress keep our mind and emotions healthy. Spiritually, we are constantly being tested—stressed—by our Creator. This "refining" is one path to improved spiritual health. I'm sure you can think of countless other examples, but my point is a simple one: Stress is not only normal—it's necessary.

However, too much stress at one single time or for too long of a time (what doctors call *chronic stress*) can lead to weakness in all four of your health wheels. Most of us are created with a capacity to handle a certain amount of stress—our "stress bucket," so to speak. Some have very small buckets and others have much larger buckets. No matter what our capacity for coping with stress is, if there's too much stress and our bucket fills, then the stress invariably spills over.

We are created to respond to stress in a variety of physical, emotional, and spiritual ways. For example, physically, when confronted with more stress than we are designed for—a large stress all at once or a smaller amount of relentless stress—our blood pressure and pulse will increase. In the short run, this is healthy; it's our body's way of getting us ready to respond. But in the long run, if this natural "fight or flight" stress response becomes our way of life, it can hurt us physically in a number of ways:

- It can damage our blood vessels and heart.
- It can cause our body to release hormones that cause the liver to release sugar (for fuel) and at the same time store fat as a backup fuel. But if we don't use that fuel source, then the fat is deposited—particularly in our abdominal region.
- It can cause our adrenal glands to "poop out." The adrenal gland is the source of adrenaline, which is one of our energy-producing hormones. If there is less of this hormone, our sleep can be disrupted and we can have decreased energy and performance during the day.
- It can cause our muscles to tense up—a good thing if we need to suddenly respond to a threat, but if it occurs chronically, it can lead to headaches, jaw pain, neck and lower back pain, and achy muscles.
- It can increase the release of stomach acid and affect the motility of the intestine and colon—leading to a variety of gastrointestinal upsets and disturbances.
- It can even suppress the immune system—possibly making us more susceptible to infections and to certain chronic illnesses.

I could go on, but you get the point: Too much stress can and will keep you from becoming a highly healthy person.

So what about you? Are there too many stressors in your life? There are several free, easy-to-use stress evaluation tools on the Internet. HealthCentral.com's "Cool Tools" can be accessed via www.highlyhealthy.net. You'll be taken to a page that will allow you to take the "Stress Management Mini-Profile," as well as the more comprehensive "Stress Test."

The twenty-five-question "Stress Management Mini-Profile" is easy to take and will report your results instantly. The results will indicate the areas in which "You're On Track" and the areas where "You Can Improve." When I took this exam (while writing this book and having just moved across the country to begin a new job), it was no surprise to receive a report showing that my stress level was critically high.

There is a classic stress measurement tool first created in 1967, known as "The Life Stress Test" or "The Holmes and Rahe Test." My rating on this test, which measures what researchers say are the most stressful life events, was even higher (indicating more stress) than my rating on the "Stress Management Mini-Profile" at HealthCentral.com.

Finally, HealthCentral's "Reduce Stress Center" can be located via www.highlyhealthy.net. Here you'll find practical advice on how to reduce stress wherever possible and manage the levels with which we all must deal.

Does stress reduction help you become a more highly healthy person? It certainly plays an important role for those who have heart disease. A study by researchers at Duke University Medical Center showed that heart patients dramatically lower their chance of having more cardiac problems by utilizing stress reduction techniques.

Duke's stress management program involved weekly sessions lasting ninety minutes. They included classroom teaching about heart disease and stress, training in stress-reduction and muscle-relaxing skills, and small group support. Ironically, according to Dr. James Blumenthal, only about 10 to 20 percent of heart patients ever wind up in these kinds of programs—probably for two reasons: (1) insurances often won't cover the treatment and (2) doctors say it is surprisingly hard to convince patients they have a stress problem, even after suffering a heart attack.

What if you choose *not* to reduce your stress levels? You may not suffer a heart attack, but untreated stress can lead to depression or other weaknesses in your emotional wheel.

Take a Stress Test

If you scored high on one of the screening tools, reducing the levels of your daily stress will contribute to your efforts to become more highly healthy.

Taking short walks—during breaks or at lunchtime—can reduce stress for most people. Whenever the weather permits, consider taking a walk with a friend or a loved one—your spouse or kids—before dinner. It's great family time, reduces stress, improves sleep, and can even reduce your appetite! My friend Rob Person calls it "taking time to kick the leaves."

Try taking "emotional wheel health breaks" every two or three hours each day. Think of something you like to do—read, journal, walk, meditate, sing, listen to music—and do it, even if only for a few minutes. Highly healthy people make taking breaks and enjoying pleasant activities a high priority!

Evaluating Anxiety

We all know what it's like to feel anxious. Do you remember the butterflies in your stomach before a first date or a big presentation to your boss, the tension you feel when someone is angry with you, the way your heart pounds when you're in danger? Anxiety, in its most basic form, is healthy—designed by our Creator to arouse us to and get us ready for action. Anxiety can prepare you physically and emotionally for a threatening situation. For me, anxiety caused me to study harder for my exams; it's what keeps me on my toes when I'm giving a speech or doing a television interview. Anxiety is designed both to help us cope and to assist us in performing at a higher level.

An *anxiety disorder* is another matter. The disorder occurs when normal anxiety does the opposite of what it was designed to do. Instead of helping you cope, it prevents you from coping and dramatically disrupts your daily life. Anxiety disorders aren't just a case of "bad nerves." They are illnesses that often have roots in both the biological makeup of the person and his or her past experiences. Not surprisingly, anxiety disorders frequently run in families.

Virtually all anxiety disorders make a person feel anxious most (or all) of the time—usually without any specific reason. For some who live with this disorder, the anxious feelings may be so uncomfortable that to avoid them they have to stop some or most of their everyday activities. For others, panic attacks can occur so swiftly and strongly that they result in experiences of terror, which can completely immobilize the individual.

Of all the disorders in the emotional wheel, anxiety disorders are the most common. Over my two decades of medical practice, the research related to mental disorders, mental health, and the brain has progressed in a dramatic fashion. Scientists are learning more and more about what anxiety disorders are, what they are caused by, and how to treat them. There are several types of anxiety disorders, each with its own distinct features and its own treatment protocol.

Many people, especially people of religious conviction, misunderstand these disorders and think that people should be able to overcome the symptoms by sheer willpower or by more faithful observance of religious ritual or practice. However, for people with these disorders, wishing them away does not work. But there is good news. There are new and revolutionary treatments that can help.

The purpose of this section is not to discuss these disorders or their treatments in depth but to convince you that if your emotional wheel is not strong, you can strengthen it. If you don't work to improve it, it is less likely that you'll become a highly healthy person. But I do want to briefly discuss the most common of the anxiety disorders—one called generalized anxiety disorder (GAD).

One of my patients on my first day of practice in the Smoky Mountains had classic GAD. "I've always been a worrier," Bill confided. "I worry about *everything!* I'm *always* keyed up, *always* on the go. Doc, I *can't* stop—it's like I'm unable to relax. At times the spells come and go, and at other times it's with me all the time. These worrying and fretting spells can go on and on. I worry about things for days at a time—getting more and more nervous and uptight the more I think about it. I just can't let some things go.

"On top of that," he added, "I'm having terrible sleep problems. I get to thinking about things at bedtime—and it's like my energy gets going. Other times I'll wake up in the middle of the night, get to thinking about things, and get so wired up I can't go back to sleep. Sometimes, when I'm having one of these spells, I'll feel light-headed. Or, worse yet, my heart starts racing or pounding and that scares me to death—and it makes me worry *even more*.

"Doc, I need you to fix me. Check out my heart—or my thyroid. Something's going on here—and it ain't good!"

So I did check Bill's heart, and I did a thorough screening of a blood sample—only to discover that all of his systems, including his thyroid, were fine. But when I asked him to take an anxiety assessment questionnaire, his scores indicated a severe anxiety disorder.

It took a second medical opinion for this man to accept the fact that virtually all of his physical symptoms were from GAD. But once he came to accept it and began to take the proper prescription medication for his condition, he showed a dramatic improvement in his emotional health. I suspected he could do even better if he would undergo some good cognitive-behavioral therapy, which is another highly recommended treatment for GAD. But Bill didn't take my advice. Like many with GAD and other mental and emotional disorders (for whom there is a stigma associated with seeing a counselor), he refused to seek counseling. Nevertheless, not only did Bill do well with the treatment he chose, but so have his three sons, all of whom have GAD.

GAD is much more than the normal anxiety people experience from day to day. It's usually lifelong and is worsened by specific stressors. Most of the time, however, nothing in particular seems to provoke it. People with GAD worry at length about health, money, job, family, or work. For many, simply the thought of getting through the day provokes anxiety. They are unable to relax and often have trouble falling asleep or staying asleep. Their worries are almost always accompanied by physical symptoms—especially trembling, twitching, muscle tension, headaches, irritability, sweating, or hot flashes. They may feel light-headed or out of breath. They may feel nauseated or have to go to the bathroom frequently. They may have palpitations or atypical chest pain. Sometimes they feel as though they have a lump in the throat. They tend to feel tired, have trouble concentrating, and sometimes suffer depression, too.

GAD usually comes on gradually. Most folks find that the symptoms start in childhood or adolescence, but it's not unusual for it to begin in adulthood or even in the senior years. GAD is more common in women than in men and often occurs in relatives. One clue that a person has this disorder is that he or she will spend at least six months worrying excessively about a number of everyday problems.

When Bill first came to see me, he was not highly healthy; over the course of time, as I taught him how to evaluate both his physical and emotional wheels, he was able to discern a significant area of weakness—an area he was willing to begin to strengthen. He did so, and I'm convinced it was an important step in becoming more highly healthy.

Check Your Emotional Wheel Pressure

If you frequently experience anxiety—and even if you don't—take the Zung Self-Rated Anxiety Scale questionnaire at my Website at www.highlyhealthy.net. If you score higher than fifty, you should see your physician or a mental health professional for further evaluation.

Other self-tests for anxiety disorders can also be found via www.highlyhealthy.net. Scoring information is available at each site.

Evaluating Depression

Depression is the second most common chronic disorder that can weaken the emotional wheel and prevent people from becoming highly healthy. It often accompanies anxiety disorders, and when it does, it needs to be treated along with the anxiety disorder. Depression is commonly accompanied by feelings of sadness, apathy, and hopelessness, as well as by changes in appetite or sleep. Depression can also make it difficult for some people to concentrate.

Thelma was in her late sixties and was the life of the small Presbyterian church in town. If the doors were open, she was there. Her family had built that church. Her love, gifts, and prayers sustained it. But slowly she began drifting away. As the pastor and elders began to notice her absences, one of the elders commented, "You know, even when she's here—well, she's not really here. She seems distant."

Several folks from her church went to Thelma's home to visit. She adamantly claimed that she had no hidden anger or unmet expectations. She just didn't feel like going out as much, now that she was "getting on." The pastor's wife insisted that she see her physician for a physical checkup. He reported that Thelma was physically fine. The exam and all the tests were reported to be normal.

After that, Thelma seemed to disappear from church. People occasionally saw her at the grocery store, but when she saw them, she'd just turn and go the other way.

Barb and I went to see her in the spring of 1982. We didn't know Thelma, but we knew her neighbor. I hadn't been in this small town very long—in fact, I'd only been in practice a few months. The neighbor was concerned. "Something's wrong with that woman," she told me. "She always decorates her house and yard for Christmas—but not this year. She always bakes for the whole neighborhood during the holidays—but not this year. But worst of all, she *always* plants a garden. This year, she hasn't even tilled!"

When I knocked on her door, Thelma opened it only a crack. We introduced ourselves, and she let us in. She tried to be sociable but just wasn't up to it. I knew what was wrong. Within minutes of entering the house, *I* felt depressed. Being around a depressed person can make you feel depressed. I asked a few diagnostic questions. She admitted she had trouble going to sleep and staying asleep. Her energy and motivation were gone. Her concentration had vanished. She felt downhearted. She confided that she'd thought about suicide, but then quickly added, "I'd *never* do that. I love my kids and grandkids too much!"

I explained to her some of the causes of depression and just how easily it could be treated. She promised to make an appointment with me that week. She did. And within just a few days of starting a simple and inexpensive treatment (a generic tricyclic antidepressant), the "old" Thelma started to bloom. By the time her corn was knee-high, she was back!

Researchers tell us that much of what manifests as depression is caused by an imbalance in the hormones of the brain. These types of depression can be fairly easily and quickly treated with a variety of treatments—modern anti-depression medications, dietary supplements, nutritional therapies, exercise, light therapy, pastoral counseling, or psychotherapy. However, a number of studies have shown that patients with depression who are treated with medication and psychotherapy (even simple counseling) almost always do better than those who receive only medication or only psychotherapy. Not only do they seem to get better faster; they stay healthier longer and have fewer relapses.

Now, to illustrate the way many of the ten essentials work together, consider the topic of treating depression with exercise. James A. Blumenthal, Ph.D., and his colleagues surprised many people in 1999 when they demonstrated that regular exercise is as effective as antidepressant medications for patients who suffer from major depression. The researchers studied 156 older adults diagnosed with major depression, assigning some to receive the antidepressant Zoloft (setraline), some to do thirty minutes of exercise three times a week, and some to participate in both treatments. According to Blumenthal,

"Our findings suggest that a modest exercise program is an effective, robust treatment for patients with major depression who are positively inclined to participate in it. The benefits of exercise are likely to endure, particularly among those who adopt it as a regular, ongoing life activity."

Recently Blumenthal's team released the results of a follow-up study. They continued to follow the same subjects for six additional months and found that the group that exercised but did not receive Zoloft did better than either of the other two groups. They also reported a very interesting finding with regard to the group that received both Zoloft and exercise. These subjects were more likely to become depressed again than were the subjects who only exercised. The researchers speculated as to why the combination group had higher depression relapse rates than the exercise-only group: "It is conceivable that the concurrent use of medication may undermine the psychological benefits of exercise." Dr. Blumenthal speculated that patients might have incorporated the belief, "I took an antidepressant and got better" instead of the more empowering belief, "I was dedicated and worked hard with the exercise program; it wasn't easy, but I beat this depression."

Will exercise work as well outside the laboratory? It depends on the person being treated. The patients in these studies appear to have been highly motivated to exercise, and the researchers would call them on the phone to remind them if they missed their exercise session. Not everybody has this level of accountability or is this motivated to make a significant lifestyle change. If you aren't *motivated* to be highly healthy, chances are you won't become highly healthy.

The bottom line is this: The vast majority of people who suffer from depression can become healthier—even highly healthy. You don't have to "put up with" chronic or disabling depression!

Depression Assessment Tools

How can you check the "pressure" in your emotional wheel—at least as far as depression is concerned? I recommend several sites on the Internet that have excellent assessment tools.

Dr. William Zung, a psychiatrist, developed the Zung Self-Rating Depression Scale screening tool. You can view and print the twenty questions and grading form by going to my Website at www.highlyhealthy.net. A score over fifty should prompt you to seriously consider seeing a physician or mental health professional.

A shorter online assessment for depression can also be found via www.highlyhealthy.net. Keep in mind that, although it's easier to take than the Zung questionnaire, it may not be as accurate. The New York University

Department of Psychiatry produced the evaluations from which this screening tool was derived.

Another depression questionnaire and additional information on depression from the National Mental Health Association can be accessed at my Website www.highlyhealthy.net.

These depression self-evaluation tools are designed to help you determine if you should see a health care professional about your feelings. These are screening tests only and should *never* replace a thorough evaluation by your physician.

Bust the Blues

Has your "get up and go" got up and gone? Is your motivation, concentration, energy, appetite, or sleep pattern abnormal or reduced? Has your interest in work or hobbies been waning? Do you feel more "blue" than in the past? If after reading this section of the book you think it's even remotely possible that you may be experiencing depression at present, take one of these self-tests today. With depression, the earlier you are diagnosed, the more quickly and successfully you can inflate your emotional health wheel.

ANTIDOTES TO A POISONOUS ATTITUDE

I hope you're beginning to have a good sense of the overall health of your emotional wheel. If you've discovered that this is one wheel that is properly inflated, then you should be motivated, based on the medical research, to continue overcoming unhealthy stress, anxiety, and depression, as well as cultivating a positive attitude and optimistic approach to problem solving.

But, you might be thinking, *I'm just a naturally sour person. I don't see what there is to be so "up" and optimistic about in this world. I couldn't have a positive outlook if my life depended on it.* Well, your excuses sound great, but they are just that—*excuses.* Let me suggest four antidotes—hope, gratitude, humor, and kindness—to confront what may be one of your biggest obstacles to being a highly healthy person, namely, your own attitude!

The Hope Antidote

Researchers have demonstrated that *how* we think and *what* we think can actually change how our brain and body function. Remaining mentally engaged with life—being a lifelong learner—not only potentially protects the brain against devastating diseases like Alzheimer's but also reflects an underlying attitude of hope and optimism about the future.

In *Living to 100: Lessons in Living to Your Maximum Potential at Any Age*, coauthor Margery Hutter Silver, Ed.D., points people to the benefits of adopting a positive attitude. In their study of some one hundred centenarians, Silver and her fellow researcher, Thomas J. Perls, M.D., M.P.H., discovered that the men and women they studied who had lived long and well had a similar positive outlook on life and on its inevitable ups and downs. (You can access their "Living to 100 Life Expectancy Calculator" via www.highlyhealthy.net, where you can take this informative self-test.) Among their findings, those who live to the age of one hundred

- handle stress well—they're very adaptable;
- seem to feel they can solve a problem, then move on; and
- have a positive attitude. Even people with physical difficulties maintained a grateful attitude and actively looked for solutions. They didn't just sit around and feel sorry for themselves.

I'd add that those who believe they have much to look forward to in life tend to enjoy better health, especially better emotional health.

I still smile when I think about two sisters I cared for in my practice in Bryson City, North Carolina. The Monteith sisters lived together for ninety-five years. Carrie's physical health was slowly declining, and as she grew sicker, she worried about her sister, Cora. I'll never forget hearing Cora tell Carrie, "Don't worry about me, girl. I've got things to do." She then enumerated a long list of projects and plans—both at home and at church. As Cora went through the list, Carrie just smiled. I could see the concern she'd been feeling for her sister dissolve as she realized that Cora would keep on living with hope and determination till her last day on earth.

Dr. David Snowden, an epidemiologist and neurology professor at the University of Kentucky, began studying aging and Alzheimer's disease among a nationwide group of elderly nuns in 1986. His most recent findings are published in what is known as the "Nun Study." Snowden found that "nuns who had articulated strong positive emotions in their early writings—using such words as 'happy,' 'joy,' 'hopeful'—lived as much as ten years longer than others." This conclusion dovetails with research on hope by C. R. Snyder, a clinical psychology professor at the University of Kansas. Snyder reported, "Hope really pays its dividends when there are stressful events in life. When something goes wrong, [high-hope people] don't conclude they're stupid or dumb, as a low-hope person would. They say, 'Hey, I didn't use the right strategy. That gives me a clue as to another way to go about this.'" Bottom line,

Snyder's research showed that people who have hopeful outlooks do better in almost all aspects of life, and they experience less stress.

But that's just not the type of person I am, you might still be protesting. *Maybe I'd be healthier if I were more hopeful and upbeat, but I'm not!* Dr. Snowden makes this encouraging comment: "I think personality drives much of the findings we reported, . . . but that doesn't mean we can't change it. It's called learning."

I couldn't agree more. The longer I practiced as a family physician, the more I was able to recognize and diagnosis an insidious killer—hopelessness! Of course, I had to first be sure the ailment wasn't caused by a physical illness—anemia, hypothyroidism, and so forth—or an emotional disruption—depression, anxiety, chronic stress. But once I ruled out these kinds of causes, nine times out of ten the source of the hopelessness wasn't what you might expect—a naturally negative personality or temperament. Rather, the source most often proved to be a flat spiritual wheel.

I'm convinced that hope—true hope—is rooted in a personal relationship with our Creator. Knowing God and pleasing him result in an abiding hope. In other words, it may be impossible to have a full and balanced emotional wheel if you have a flat spiritual one.

The writer of the Old Testament book of Ecclesiastes makes this profound statement:

> A man can do nothing better than to eat and drink and find satisfaction in his work. This too, I see, is from the hand of God, for without him, who can eat or find enjoyment? To the man who pleases him, God gives wisdom, knowledge and happiness, but to the sinner he gives the task of gathering and storing up wealth to hand it over to the one who pleases God. This too is meaningless, a chasing after the wind.

If you're feeling hopeless, is there any hope that hope can be found? Most assuredly! We can see a glimpse of true hope in this ancient passage of Hebrew wisdom, for it is *God* who gives wisdom, knowledge, and happiness to the person who pleases him. Where are meaning and purpose and hope found? According to the writer of Ecclesiastes, only in pleasing God—our Creator.

Blaise Pascal, the French physicist and philosopher, wrote: "There is a God-shaped vacuum in the heart of every man which cannot be filled by any created thing, but only by God the Creator." Samuel Smiles wrote, "Hope is the companion of power, and mother of success; for who so hopes strongly has within him the gift of miracles." Hope is healing, and one cannot be highly healthy without the hope antidote—which springs first and foremost from a personal relationship with God.

If you're still searching for satisfaction and for hope, you may be trying to fill the "God-shaped vacuum" of your soul with other things. In my experience, people who do this only find dead-end streets. Eventually they lose heart—lose hope. And people without hope inevitably lack satisfaction and joy. As a result, they're simply not able to become and stay highly healthy.

Wayne was one of my most hopeless patients. I was his family physician for nearly fifteen years. I delivered their three children and cared for his wife, Sharon, during two miscarriages. I grew to love them as patients, but I was disturbed by Wayne's caustic hopelessness, which manifested itself in a pervasive pessimism. No matter what I told him, no matter how I cajoled or coaxed, he couldn't—or wouldn't—crawl out of his self-imposed "slough of despond." His hopeless outlook—the result of a flat spiritual wheel—affected his physical, emotional, and relational wheels in numerous negative ways.

Wayne had grown up in church and had always been active in church programs. Yet, as I got to know him better I became convinced that, although Wayne knew church, he did not know God—at least not in a personally meaningful way.

One day we went to lunch together. I let Wayne know that my life journey had been similar to his. I, too, had grown up in church. I was good at religion (humankind's best attempt to find God). But during childhood I had never gotten to know God intimately. I told Wayne that I was in college before I began to deeply understand the fact that God loved me more than I could imagine and that he desired a personal relationship with me. It was my selfishness and my wrongdoing, I explained, that kept me separated from God.

"Wayne," I asked, "do you believe that God *wants* to know you—to have a relationship with you?"

I was surprised, but delighted, when he silently nodded yes.

"Do you have that type of relationship with him now?" I asked.

He shook his head no, and tears began to fill his eyes.

"How about starting today?"

He smiled and nodded.

Then we prayed together—right there in Denny's! On that day, a highly religious man—a man who had never really known God personally and whose emotional and spiritual wheels were flat—chose a new route on the way to becoming highly healthy. That day was the start of a new life, a new commitment to live with eternity in view. It was the kindling of a profound hope for Wayne. As his relationship with God grew, his emotional and spiritual wheels became filled and balanced—followed by improvements in his relational and physical wheels.

I recommended that Wayne meet with his pastor to discuss strategies for improving his spiritual health. He did so. As Wayne began to grow spiritually, his pessimism and hopelessness began to dissolve. Sharon told me, "He's a new man. He's actually fun to be around!"

When I left my practice in Florida, Wayne and Sharon and their kids were highly healthy. With the demise of hopelessness came health.

Knowing God—Not Just Knowing about Him

Do you know God in a personal way? If you're not sure, I encourage you to call a pastor at a local Bible-believing church and schedule an appointment to talk. You'll find that most pastors will be delighted to talk to you—without pressuring you!

If you do know God personally, if you possess this critical relationship, then where are your priorities right now? Are you bored with life? With your job? With your spouse or friends? With your hobbies? With your church? With your relationship with God? Perhaps other pursuits have dulled your passion for spending time in God's presence and serving him. Where is your meaning and purpose? In money, pleasure, power, position, relationships? Simply put, all of these things must find their proper perspective in a life devoted to the number one priority, namely, *pleasing God*. If your priorities seem to have gotten out of whack, schedule a visit with your pastor to talk—soon! You need encouragement to regain the hope you've lost.

The Gratitude Antidote

There are many ways to develop a positive attitude, but one easy way to begin is with the habit of giving thanks. One recent Thanksgiving Day Barb and I sat around the table after a glorious dinner with a small group of family and friends. One of our friends, who was like a daughter to us, asked if we could practice a tradition her family had enjoyed for generations. "We just go around in a circle," Ellen explained, "telling each other what we're thankful for. Each time you speak, you can only share *one* thing. We just keep going around for as long as it takes."

I smiled. *This probably won't take very long.* Boy, was I mistaken. Ellen began. "Today I am grateful for a new 'family' with which I can share this special holiday."

The next person in the circle continued. "Today I am grateful for a job that I love."

"Today I am grateful for pumpkin pie and ice cream," said the next person.

"Today I am grateful for a warm home and a loving husband."

To my amazement, this simple exercise continued over forty-five minutes, bringing much joy and laughter. As we cleared the table, you could hear individuals whistling or humming to themselves. Attitudes were positive—indeed, jolly.

We could have complained or gossiped or discussed our ills and problems; we could have concentrated on the difficult times our country has experienced—all of which would have most certainly depressed us. But Ellen chose to demonstrate the age-old principle that an attitude of gratitude almost always generates positive feelings and a sense of well-being.

Frederic and Mary Ann Brussat observe, "Writer G. K. Chesterton had the right idea when he said we need to get in the habit of 'taking things with gratitude and not taking things for granted.' Gratitude puts everything in a fresh perspective; it enables us to see the many blessings all around us. And the more ways we find to give thanks, the more things we find to be grateful for. Giving thanks takes practice, however. We get better at it over time."

One good way to develop an attitude of gratitude is to begin a gratitude list or a gratitude journal—a practice endorsed by Oprah Winfrey and popularized by Sarah Ban Breathnach's best-seller *Simple Abundance*. In fact, this concept is so well accepted that a 1998 Gallup poll showed that more than 90 percent of Americans believe that expressing gratitude makes them happy.

I gave one of my patients who had a particularly bad attitude (and the chronic depression that often goes with it) the assignment of keeping a daily gratitude journal for two weeks. On her next visit, she said, "I can't believe how much better it makes me feel and function. I still have bad moods and disappointments—but they seem to be getting better by the day. On days when I keep a list of all the little things that give me a lift, it's amazing how the good feelings just grow. On days when I forget—well, my bad attitude gets the best of me!"

Behavioral psychologists have taken note of the ageless principle that an attitude of gratitude will increase feelings of optimism and well-being. Psychology professors Michael McCullough, Ph.D., and Bob Emmons, Ph.D., have performed several studies on the perspectives and dimensions of gratitude. Specifically, they've examined whether the positive attitudes that come from giving thanks can ease the emotional burdens and stress of women with breast cancer and people with neuromuscular disorders. It should be no surprise that the early results are positive—so much so that McCullough hosted the first-ever conference on gratitude's positive health effects.

In one of the studies, researchers asked one group of volunteers to keep a daily log of their five most irritating hassles of the day. A second group spent time each day listing five ways in which they thought they were better off than their peers. A third group wrote daily about five things for which they were grateful that day. All three groups also kept a daily record of their moods and physical health. At the end of three weeks, the people who kept gratitude lists reported having greater energy, fewer health complaints, and more overall feelings of wellbeing than those who complained or gloated each day, according to results published in the spring 2000 issue of the *Journal of Social and Clinical Psychology.*

Professors McCullough and Emmons have continued to publish their findings about the impact of gratitude on helping people achieve high degrees of health. In four studies they've examined the relationship between one's health and one's level of gratitude. In another study they've shown that selfratings and observer ratings of the grateful disposition are associated with positive effect and well-being (an improved emotional wheel), improved social behaviors and traits (an improved relational wheel), and improvements in measures of religiousness/spirituality (an improved spiritual wheel).

They were able to replicate these findings in a large, nonstudent sample. A third study revealed similar results and provided evidence that as gratitude increases, the negative emotions of envy and a materialistic attitude decrease. They demonstrated that this is true whether one is an extrovert or an introvert or whether one is naturally positive or negative.

Researchers believe that an active cultivation of gratitude results in positive attitudes and well-being because of the principles of *cognitive therapy* (a form of psychotherapy that helps people replace negative explanations of events with more positive ones). When you find yourself brooding over an unpleasant experience, for instance, you can consciously *choose* to find a reason to be grateful. By doing so, you perform your own spontaneous cognitive therapy.

In two studies undertaken in the late 1990s, psychology professors Barbara Fredrickson, Ph.D., and Robert W. Levenson, Ph.D., caused anxiety or fear in a group of subjects by first showing them disturbing film clips and then showed clips intended to cause contentment, amusement, or other positive emotions. The films that triggered positive feelings helped participants recover from negative emotions faster than did sad or disturbing films. Here's the conclusion: Positive emotions may actually neutralize harmful ones. "It may be easier," said Dr. Fredrickson, "for people to cultivate mirth, gratitude, and other positive states than to struggle to banish negative feelings like sadness and anger."

Due to the publicity generated by Oprah and others in the media, the public isn't waiting for scientists to explain why gratitude works. People are simply beginning en masse to keep gratitude lists. Why? A simple five-minute daily gratitude ritual makes believers out of many. It's like taking an emotional aspirin on emotionally painful days. I've seen a growing understanding among professionals and laypeople that it's not life events that make a person happy or unhappy; it's how a person copes with those events that makes the difference. Or, as my granddad used to say, "Walt, if you're not content with what you have, you'll never be content with what you want!"

Keeping a gratitude journal is something most people have to work at over time. Researchers observe that it's not a natural tendency for most people, but that with time it can become automatic. Yet, isn't that true for all of the essentials of highly healthy people? They are *not* automatic. They take effort. You need to determine whether your health—and that of your loved ones—is worth the effort.

The more you cultivate a positive coping style, the more likely you are to demonstrate feelings of well-being and happiness, no matter what your lot in life.

Take an Emotional Aspirin and Call Me in the Morning

When you begin to dwell on or complain about a bad event or situation in your life, you can consciously turn the thought or self-talk around. Just tell yourself, "Now tell me something good."

Try this experiment: Start taking an "emotional aspirin" every day for a week. Keep a small journal at your bedside. Each night before going to sleep, record five things for which you are grateful. Then, for a minute or two, reflect on each item you recorded and thank God for the gifts you've been given. See what happens to your feelings over the course of just a few days.

Here's another experiment you can try: The next time something bad or irritating or disappointing happens to you—or the next time you find yourself brooding over an unpleasant experience—*stop yourself.* Choose instead—right away—to find a reason to be grateful. Don't be surprised to find your attitude change instantly!

The Humor Antidote

In *Living to 100,* the authors note that the centenarians they studied have a wonderful sense of humor. Indeed, a great deal of medical research has demonstrated the direct impact that laughter has on boosting both the immune and cardiovascular systems.

I can still hear Leonard's contagious laugh and see his face. He was nearing ninety-two when he walked into my office on my first day of practice. "Been looking for a younger doctor," he stated bluntly. "I find that younger doctors keep me younger. 'Sides, some of the old codgers 'round here don't have no sense of humor!"

Our relationship was off to a great start. Leonard became not only one of my favorite patients but also a dear friend to our family. His list of physical maladies was not brief. He suffered from a severe form of heart failure—the result of several heart attacks suffered through the years. With even mild exertion, he'd experience chest pain. He also had a chronic, irritating dermatitis, couldn't see or hear very well, and was crippled with arthritis worsened by injuries from a number of logging accidents from his youth. Yet the time I spent with him, whether in the office or around town, was always a time filled with laughter. Leonard knew more good jokes than any man I'd met before—or since.

Leonard had a high "humor quotient." His ability and willingness to laugh, to lighten his load, was part of the reason I considered Leonard highly healthy—in spite of his physical problems.

Medical research has documented in a number of ways the essential of humor in highly healthy people. Researchers at the University of Maryland tested the "ability to laugh" of several hundred patients. Those with the lowest "humor quotient" were significantly more likely to have heart disease. In fact, they were 40 percent less likely to laugh at the "gaffes, mix-ups, and irritations" of day-to-day life than were those without heart disease.

While presenting this study at the November 2000 meeting of the American Heart Association, Michael Miller, M.D., said, "Laughter is no substitute for eating properly, exercising, and controlling blood pressure and cholesterol with medication, if need be, but enjoying a few laughs every day couldn't hurt, and our research suggests that it might help your heart health."

How does laughter work? The studies I've reviewed don't provide a conclusive answer. Nevertheless, many researchers feel that lightening one's emotional load through laughter causes the body to decrease the level of inflammation in the walls of the blood vessels—an inflammation that seems to contribute to hardening of the arteries, heart attacks, heart failure, and strokes. When the inflammation is reduced through laughing, the risk of blood clots decreases, as does blood pressure.

Researchers at Marywood University in Scranton, Pennsylvania, showed that students would have a significant rise in their blood pressure and heart rate prior to giving a speech in front of the class. Yet the students who watched a funny television program (which caused them to laugh hysterically) before they gave their speech had much lower elevations in their heart rate and blood pressure while delivering their talk. It was as though the comedy "inoculated" the students against the negative effects of anxiety and stress.

A physician friend told me how stressed he'd feel during busy days of seeing patients back to back. One weekend he decided to purchase a small television set with a videotape recorder built in. Before the workweek began, he rented three comedy videos and brought them to the office with him. He watched part of a video while eating lunch. His laughter was so loud that his nurse checked on him. In no time, she and other staff members joined him for lunch and videos. "My stress levels dropped like a brick," my friend told me. "And not only mine, but my staff's as well! We began handling the stress of the day without getting more stressed ourselves. And we seemed to provide even better care for our patients who were suffering from stress."

Laughter Is the Best Prescription

Down through the years I've consistently written a couple of different notes on prescription pads for my patients who are a bit too serious. Consider filling both of these prescriptions for immediate relief!

Learn to laugh at yourself. When you goof up, do you get mad? When you accidentally drop something, do you get angry, or even curse at yourself? Being a perfectionist, I suffered from this problem for a long time. But I'm learning to lower my expectations of myself—to laugh at myself. I'm convinced I'm healthier for it. I've learned that slipups and less-than-perfect behavior are part of everyone's daily life as a human being. Now I laugh at myself when I put a box of cereal in the refrigerator or the milk in the pantry. I chuckle when I misplace my glasses—which means I'm laughing throughout the day! These goof-ups have become an opportunity to raise my humor quotient rather than an occasion to belittle myself.

Become an expert at giggling. Take several doses of giggles every day. Chuckle, cackle, chortle, and belly-laugh your way to higher degrees of health. You need only be a student of yourself. What are some things that make you giggle? It may be a funny video, a humorous book, or even a few choice comics in the daily newspaper. One of my partners in family practice had a collection of desk calendars—daily jokes, funny medical stories, Gary Larson cartoons. Every hour or two, my colleague would turn the page to that day in one of the calendars and enjoy a giggle. He loved sharing them with me—and with his patients, too.

The Kindness Antidote

At least one leading psychologist believes that kindness is contagious and that witnessing good deeds not only makes you feel better emotionally but can inspire you to model that behavior yourself. Jonathan Haidt, Ph.D., psychology professor at the University of Virginia, asserts that witnessing selfless acts of kindness or generosity can cause an actual physical sensation—something akin to a fluttering heart or a tingling feeling all over one's body. That sensation, Haidt believes, "is neither an inconsequential response limited to one transitory moment of awe, nor a vague and indecipherable 'feeling.' Rather, the effect that comes from witnessing acts of charity or courage may be a profoundly important universal phenomenon worthy of scientific research."

Dr. Haidt is a pioneer in studying the effect that kindness—good deeds and acts of valor—has on those who witness it. He calls the positive effect *elevation*. I like to think of it as pumping air into a flat emotional wheel. While experts caution that Haidt's work is still largely theoretical, I believe we can apply this principle of elevation in everyday interactions with our friends, family members, and colleagues.

One of my favorite books is William Bennett's *The Book of Virtues*, which describes many examples of virtuous behavior from the libraries of world history and famous literature. Bennett calls these examples "a potent source of moral exemplars for kindness and virtuous behavior." According to Bennett, virtuous behavior not only benefits the observer in particular and society in general, but it also benefits the person who models the kindness or virtue. According to Dr. Haidt and Dr. Bennett, kindness—both receiving it *and* giving it—literally results in higher degrees of personal health.

Medical reporter Mark Moran points out, "The study of elevation by Haidt is part of a larger movement termed 'positive psychology.' It is a growing area of scientific inquiry focusing on aspects of human experience once considered off-limits to scientists: forgiveness, spirituality, gratitude, optimism, humor. [These are all aspects that are essential to becoming highly healthy!] In part, this movement is a reaction to a long tradition within the psychological sciences of concentrating on what's wrong with an individual rather than on what's right."

So how might these insights be put to use in our lives? Dr. Haidt notes that the principles of elevation are already at work in a school-based education program called "Kindness Is Contagious: Catch It." This program, which began in a single Kansas City, Missouri, school, has since spread to more than 400 public schools. Among the activities the program encourages is one called "Pass It On," in which a teacher provides an overview of what kindness is, and then looks for a spontaneous act of kindness among his or her students. After witnessing such an act, the teacher gives the kind child an apple, for example. The child then becomes a witness and must pass the apple on to someone who does a similar act of kindness. "The feedback we got was amazing," says SuEllen Fried, founder of the Stop Violence Coalition, which sponsors "Kindness Is Contagious." "Kids *wanted* to be observed performing acts of kindness."

Dave Simmons had been an All-American middle linebacker at Georgia Tech who went on to play professional football. After his football career ended, Dave began a summer camp for kids. I served as a counselor there for two summers. He poured his life into the campers and into us counselors. Dave taught that the only love that counts is *love in action.*

Dave told me about an evening when he took his daughter and son shopping. The shopping center housed a small petting zoo and some kiddie rides. The kids wanted to ride on a small train circling the zoo, so Dave gave them each a quarter and told them to enjoy the ride while he stopped in at one last store.

After emerging from the store and coming back to the ride, he saw his daughter on the train with several other children. But Brandon, his son, was standing there watching—and grinning like crazy.

"Why aren't you riding the train, Brandon?" Dave asked.

Brandon looked up at his dad, still smiling, and said, "It cost fifty cents to ride, so I gave Helen my quarter."

Then he looked over at his sister and quoted a lesson he had been taught many times by his dad: "Love is action."

As you can imagine, Dave was both stunned by Brandon's generosity and immensely proud of this small boy's virtue. Even though Dave had several quarters in his pocket, he wisely kept them there, put his arm around his son, and allowed Brandon to enjoy the benefits of love in action.

You see, Dave knew instinctively what the research is now showing: Acts of kindness provide emotional, relational, spiritual, and even physical health benefits.

Dispense a Purposeful Act of Kindness

Think of someone with whom you don't spend much time—yet someone you see often. It might be a neighbor or a colleague at work or school. Think of something you could give him or do for him—some way you could serve her or help her. Don't wait to be asked. Just do it. It won't be a "random" act of kindness but a *purposeful* one. Then go a step further and consider how you might show love in action to that person once a week.

Watch what happens to him or her—and to you!

Is all of this beginning to make sense? Are the many puzzle pieces of health beginning to come together? Are you learning how the physical and emotional health wheels really do work in unison?

Next is the *relational* wheel. It runs in tandem with the physical and emotional wheels. In fact, researchers point out that those who are optimistic or hopeful or who practice kindness and gratitude also tend to be more social, more relational. Having a healthy relational wheel is crucial to becoming a highly healthy person.

CHAPTER SEVEN

Avoid Loneliness

The Essential of Relationships

Being a doctor in a small town in the Great Smoky Mountains of western North Carolina means not only are you a family physician, you also serve as the coroner. And Bryson City was the "real" world of rural medicine. I quickly learned there were many things a doctor needed to know in practice that hadn't been taught in medical school.

One evening a sheriff's deputy called. "Doc, we got a home death we need you to come see."

At that time in North Carolina, if someone didn't die in a medical facility, the coroner had to be called to the scene, just to be sure there was no foul play. So I left our home on Hospital Hill and drove up Deep Creek Valley.

The old ramshackle home was located on a dirt road just up "Toot Holler." Two Swain County sheriff cars and the county ambulance were parked perilously at the edge of the road—leaning menacingly toward the small creek ten feet below.

I parked—in the middle of the road—and walked up to the house. The deputy met me at the door.

"Doc, sure looks natural. Ol' Lady Smith's been up here, all alone, for years. Never left the house. Never had any visitors. Never went to the doctor—not that I blame her."

He rather suspiciously examined the town's newest doctor as I ducked to enter the undersized door, ignoring his affront to the medical profession. He followed me, continuing his soliloquy. "She had a friend who brought her food and supplies. Her friend found her here this evening and called us."

And there she was. Porcelainlike skin, white and smooth. Surprisingly few wrinkles for someone born fifty-two years earlier. I suspected she saw very little sunlight in her days. She was stone-cold and stiff as a board. Rigor mortis had set in.

There was no sign of foul play. No indication of a struggle or seizure. By all outward signs she had died quietly, peacefully. As I examined her, I ran through possible causes of death in my mind. Heart attack? Heart irregularity? Infection? Stroke? Brain hemorrhage? Poisoning? All were possible, but only an autopsy could tell for sure. As I was contemplating the possibilities, the deputy lobbed a theory I hadn't considered.

"I'll tell ya what she done died of, Doc," he began slowly, almost thoughtfully. "This here woman died of loneliness." He stood there looking down at the body, rubbing his chin whiskers. "You can put whatever you want on that death certificate, but I'll tell you what, son, she done died of loneliness. I see it all the time."

He turned and walked out.

The autopsy results arrived at my office the next week. The conclusion? Mrs. Smith had arteriosclerosis (hardening of the arteries) and early coronary artery disease, stones in her gallbladder, fibroids in her uterus, and benign tumors in both of her breasts. There were signs in her brain of mini-strokes, and her teeth were in poor shape. But there was no obvious cause of death. No evidence of a massive stroke or heart attack or poisoning or infection. The pathologist declared it to be a natural death. I guessed that the medical cause of death was cardiac arrhythmia—her heart had developed an abnormal and irregular beat that would prove to be fatal.

Now, more than twenty years later, I think the deputy may have been right. Researchers have stated that loneliness is one of the leading causes of death in the United States and a major risk factor for heart disease. An increasing number of well-designed studies involving hundreds of thousands of people around the world are concluding that loneliness not only hurts us physically, emotionally, and spiritually, but it can actually kill.

Love, social support, intimacy, security, safety, satisfaction, connectedness, and community—these terms all relate to a common theme in the medical literature. It just makes sense. When we feel loved, nurtured, appreciated, valued, cared for, and supported, we are much more likely to be happier and healthier. People who avoid loneliness have a much lower risk of getting sick, and if they do become ill, they have a much greater chance of surviving. If you want to become a highly healthy person, then the simple fact is that *your relationships matter.* And they matter a lot.

God understood the problems that can result from being alone. In the first book of the Bible we are told, "God formed the man from the dust of the ground and breathed into his nostrils the breath of life, and the man became a living being." Several verses later, God said, "It is not good for the man to be alone."

The Hebrew word *lebad*, translated "alone," carries overtones of separation and even alienation, a sense of being incomplete—even a sense that the alone (lonely) person is *unable* to be complete. It connotes being apart from someone or something essential. Many Hebrews, both ancient and modern, consider aloneness as the opposite of authentic living. To them, living requires positive social relationships in family and in community. True life is not individual, it's social; it's living with others.

This ancient record of wisdom is now being proven by modern research. The kind of separateness referred to in the biblical text is a form of disease, and we now know from medical studies that loneliness can cause psychiatric disorders and mental breakdowns, and even illness and premature death. The Hebrew mind-set was that human beings truly live only insofar as they are related within their environment to others with whom they share life and love—with whom they serve God, family, and community.

But you couldn't tell that to Sam Cunningham. Sam was a loner—and like most loners, he tended to be angry, hostile, and cynical. And alone—very alone.

The ambulance brought Sam into the emergency room at Swain County Hospital. The couple that lived next door to Sam had begun to notice an unpleasant smell coming from his place. The Millers normally didn't bother Sam. He didn't seem friendly, never returned any kindness they offered—even when they'd leave a small vase of flowers at his door or one of Mrs. Miller's delicious pies. Sam never sent a thank-you note to the Millers, and he would return the vase or dishes to their front porch without even washing them. On the rare occasions when he and the Millers would actually see each other, Sam would only sneer or grunt at their greetings. So they were reluctant to go next door—but the smell compelled them.

After they had knocked for the fifth time, Sam finally opened the door. Both his appearance and his odor were horrid. He was confused and disheveled. His foot was wrapped in a rag—but soaked with putrid pus. Sam seemed to stare past them. Then he began to laugh strangely—and suddenly he slammed the door. The Millers called 911, which brought both the sheriff and an ambulance in minutes.

Sam was obese and filthy. He was what doctors call "chronically dirty." Every wrinkle had the rankest grime at its base. His toenails were thickened, long, and curled under, and his toe webs were nasty. But his right big toe was the worst. It was gangrenous.

Sam was delusional, probably from the infection that was spreading through his body. His blood pressure and blood sugar were both way off. We worked fast and hard to stabilize him, but his diseases beat us to the finish line.

"Code Blue, Emergency Room!" was announced over the hospital public-address system while I was looking at Sam's X rays in the radiology department. I sprinted to the ER. His heart had started to fibrillate, beating rapidly and erratically, and then he had a seizure. We did CPR for quite some time—but to no avail.

When I filled out his death certificate, I wrote that the cause of death was a heart attack exacerbated by obesity, hypertension, arteriosclerosis, tobacco abuse, alcoholism, diabetes, sepsis, and gangrene. But if truth be told, Sam died of loneliness.

Sam, at the age of twenty-nine, was a pathological loner. He was an extreme example of the negative separateness referred to by the ancient Hebrews. I tell his story to drive home the point that loneliness can kill.

I'm not talking about people who are natural introverts—who get their energy from being able to spend time thinking and reading alone. By and large, healthy introverts understand, enjoy, and appreciate close relationships. I'm talking instead about people who fail to realize that, unless they intentionally cultivate significant and healthy relationships, they are increasing their risk of becoming ill. Highly healthy people avoid loneliness like the plague.

Ginny, who at the age of seventy-nine is sharp, energetic, and the bargain shopper of the century, is always on the go—to the market or the mall. Her closets are overflowing with great buys she "just couldn't pass up"—even though she's lived alone for nearly two decades and will never be able to use up the forty boxes of sandwich bags stashed in the storage room. Buying small gifts for her extended family members is a favorite activity—and her kids and grandkids appreciate her generosity. But Ginny is lonely.

Ginny and her husband moved from base to base in his long army career, raised five children, and reveled in their close-knit family life. But the kids grew up and left home to start their own families. Ginny's husband died unexpectedly at the age of sixty-one. And Ginny, instead of finding purpose and enjoyment in her new life, has spent the last eighteen years trying to recapture her past. Most of her children are in their fifties and her first great-grandchild has just been born. Yet Ginny continues to be one thing and one thing only: a mother. She worries herself sick over what might happen to one of her "kids," and she spends almost every hour of her day focusing her energy on being a "mother," a role her family has for decades begged her to shed.

Even though she stays active and claims to have strong religious faith, Ginny adamantly refuses to be involved in any other relationships beyond those with family members, who can't possibly spend the kind of time with her that she has available to fill. Instead of making new friends or volunteering her many skills and personal charms in service to church or community, she chooses day after sad day to spend most of her time alone—pining for the company of her "kids."

Ginny complains about not feeling well, alluding frequently to the "fact" that she is not long for this world. But Ginny's medical checkups have always indicated a normal degree of physical health for her age. She could easily have another ten or even twenty years of vibrant life ahead of her—if she would only *choose* this option! But instead of truly living, I'm concerned that she is slowly dying of a silent killer—loneliness. If the research can be trusted, she'll simply not live as long—or as well—as she could by choosing to avoid loneliness, choosing to find warm and meaningful relationships within her community. Her children, as is appropriate and healthy, have moved on—with their spouses and loved ones. Ginny, unfortunately, is stuck in the past.

THE POWER OF HUMAN CONNECTION

Unlike Ginny, most people are aware of the need for friends and social support. In a book of daily reflections, Episcopal Bishop Edmond Lee Browning writes this:

> Community is in short supply these days. We long for it—invent small towns that never existed, put them in television shows, and wish with all our hearts that we lived in them. We want fellowship. Where I live, most of the bookstores are now also coffee bars, and people actually go there with each other on dates. We are aware of our own aloneness.

Contemporary American researcher George Barna, whose marketing research company has been providing information and analysis regarding cultural trends since 1984, concurs:

> Overall, the research paints a portrait of a nation whose adults keep themselves occupied so they do not have to face significant short-comings. . . . Many people admit to lacking relational connections and meaning in life. Those two factors are critical to gaining joy and fulfillment in life. The common solution is to keep busy and to stimulate ourselves with a variety of new experiences—that way we are not so likely to feel the pain of those fundamental holes in our life. People have discovered that if they fill the gaps with commitments and excitement, then they're less prone to feel the emptiness of loneliness and aimlessness. Of course, that just prolongs the inner despair that eventually cannot be suppressed any longer.

Over the last few decades medical research has expanded our knowledge of the importance of positive relationships and socialization on our mental, physical, and spiritual health. The verdict seems clear: People who do not regularly enjoy meaningful personal relationships with God or others—or who are in relationships devoid of love or caring—are highly likely to have lower levels of health. Lonely people are at greater risk for heart attack, heart failure, ulcers, stroke, infectious diseases, mental illness, diabetes, many types of cancer, lung disease, autoimmune disorders, and other life-threatening illnesses.

Why would this be? There are a number of explanations found in medical research.

One study (of almost 12,000 individuals) examined Japanese men who lived in Japan and compared them to Japanese men who had moved to Hawaii or California. The researchers looked at smoking, diet, exercise, cholesterol levels, and social support (the maintenance of social networks and family and community ties). The group with the lowest social support (the California group) had a threefold to fivefold increase in heart disease. The researchers concluded that social networks and close family ties help protect against disease and premature death.

Researchers at the University of Texas evaluated patients who had undergone open-heart surgery. They found that those who lacked regular activity in organized social groups—a flat relational wheel—had a fourfold increase in the risk of death. Those who reported that they did not draw strength from their religion—a flat spiritual wheel—were three times more likely to die within six months after surgery. However, these risks were additive, as those who did not engage in organized social activity *and* who did not draw strength from their religion—flat relational *and* spiritual wheels—were more than *seven* times as likely to die within six months of their surgery.

Other research has shown a strong association between lack of social support and low HDL cholesterol levels. HDL cholesterol is known as the good—or healthy—cholesterol that seems to protect the heart. Lonely people tend to have very low levels of HDL cholesterol that are not explained by diet, physical exercise, alcohol abuse, age, menopause, or smoking. Swedish researchers have shown that women who have low levels of social support have more severe disease in their coronary arteries.

Many social science researchers are now saying that, apart from our genetics, the most powerful across-the-board factor in predicting premature death and disease is lack of social support. Researchers have looked at a variety of relationship measures, such as a sense of being accepted and loved by others and a sense that the support or help of others is available. Almost all these medical studies conclude that social support affects health positively. People who believe that no one really cares for them, who don't feel close to anyone, or who feel they have no one in whom to confide or to help them out of a bind—these folks are *three to five times* as likely to experience premature death or disease.

Some studies indicate that the risk is even higher. One of the reasons is that a lonely person is more likely to practice unhealthy habits—such as abusing tobacco, alcohol, food, or drugs—but this accounts for only a portion of their risk. Anger, depression, high-stress jobs, low socioeconomic status, and lack of social support often go hand in hand with the avoidable tragedy of loneliness. When these risk factors come together in one person, their effects are compounded and can be explosively dangerous to one's health.

The good news: Reducing loneliness by developing and enhancing friendships will help improve your overall health. You don't need a large group of friends; a small group will do. Even one or two very close friends with whom you share interests and affection can do the trick.

Alan saw me every year for a physical exam. On one of these visits, he shared briefly about the rotten weekend he'd had. A colleague—someone who'd been his good friend for more than twenty years—had sent him an e-mail "bomb," a mean-spirited missile that sent Alan into a tailspin. (Modern technology has made it easier than ever to keep people more closely and regularly connected, but some folks use it to avoid intimacy rather than to enhance it.)

Alan didn't share all the details of the message, but he did describe how he handled the aftermath. At first, he felt angry. But that defense mechanism quickly gave way to a deep sense of hurt and shame, even though most of what was in the e-mail message was bluster that should have been ignored. And Alan knew it.

"I found myself becoming almost physically paralyzed as I stared at my computer screen," he told me. "My intestines felt like they were literally tying knots in my gut, and I suddenly realized I wasn't even breathing. I felt mortified. I just wanted the floor to open up so I could drop through and hide for the next ten years!" he said with a rueful grin.

Alan moped for a good twenty-four hours. He berated himself and composed retorts to Thomas in his mind until he drove himself nearly crazy. He didn't answer the phone. Bad dreams plagued him when he finally fell asleep that night. By the next day, Alan knew he was sinking fast and needed a lifeline. He recognized his old habit of isolating himself when he felt hurt and overwhelmed. He'd spent many a lonely hour in this self-imposed prison in the past; he didn't want to repeat that now. He also remembered what had helped him in the past. Even though he's a *very* busy person, he took time to tend to his own health. He took a brisk walk in a nearby park. As he walked along a path in the park, breathing in clean, fresh air, he began to feel cleansed and free, able to enjoy the beautiful day.

Alan knew what else he had to do to stay highly healthy, too. He picked up the phone. "I swear it weighed 600 pounds," he chuckled. He dialed the number of a friend he could trust—someone whose advice was always wise and good. They talked about the situation and Alan's reaction. Their conversation was warm and meaningful, and within ten minutes Alan was back on healthy ground! He'd kicked shame out of his heart and loneliness out of his world. He'd reconnected.

If Alan had chosen to keep that hurt to himself—to use loneliness as a defense, to *not* seek the comfort and advice of a longtime friend and confidant—he would have continued the downward spiral alone, and his health would have suffered.

Find a Friend

Avoid loneliness like the plague by intentionally involving yourself in a variety of positive and healthy social relationships with people you like and admire—and who are willing and able to care about you and for you.

Talk to your pastor or friends. Try different people and social situations. If you are uncomfortable after one try, shake the dust off your sandals and try another. You may be surprised how quickly you'll find individuals or a group with whom you can get along.

One tip—don't expect them to do all the giving. The more you give to your friend(s) and social groups, the more you'll get in return.

THE PARENT-CHILD BOND

Even though Ginny's health and even her life expectancy may be negatively affected by her unwillingness to reach outside her family for connection, she certainly understood something important during the years when her children were young: A loving parent is critical to a child's well-being. Researchers found that children raised in single-parent or abusive homes are significantly less healthy than those raised in families with a loving mother and father. It's not surprising to learn that healthy patterns of social caring begin early in childhood. Those of us who are blessed to have been raised in healthy two-parent families seem to reap long-term benefits. Barb and I both were raised by parents who gave us their all and are still loving each other after more than fifty years of marriage. Based on the scientific research, their relationship with each other and with us should improve our health.

In the 1950s, Harvard researchers randomly chose 126 healthy men and administered a questionnaire dealing with how they felt about their parents. Thirty-five years later, the men's medical records were reviewed. The results were stunning. Of the men who did not perceive themselves as having had a warm relationship with their mothers, 91 percent had been diagnosed with a serious disease, such as coronary artery disease, high blood pressure, duodenal ulcers, or alcoholism. The same was true in only 45 percent of those who reported a warm relationship with their mom.

Of the study participants who reported poor relationships with their dads, 82 percent had disease as compared with only 50 percent of those men who had close relationships with their dads. The most astonishing finding was that this effect was additive. *All* of the men who rated their relationship with both mom and dad as low in warmth and closeness had been diagnosed with diseases— whereas only 47 percent of those who rated their relationship with both parents as warm and intimate had disease.

Based on this research, growing up in a loving family where you feel warm and close toward both your mother and father increases your chance of being a highly healthy person. The researchers concluded that "the perception of love itself . . . may turn out to be a core . . . buffer, reducing the negative impact of stressors and pathogens and promoting immune function and healing."

Other studies reveal similar findings. In the 1940s researchers developed a "Closeness to Parents" scale and administered it to healthy students. Fifty years later the participants' medical records were examined. Students who subsequently developed cancer were significantly more likely to have reported a lack of closeness with their parents. Amazingly, the researchers showed that the predictive value of this scale did not diminish over time. In this study, those most likely to end up with cancer were those who reported the lowest score on the father-son scale.

Men and women who choose to spend most of their time at work and little or no time with their children often don't understand how harmful their actions can be to their children's health. Although most of these parents sincerely believe that the money this extra work brings in will be of benefit to their children, the benefits pale in comparison to the benefits from the time parents give to their kids. I've often told my patients that quality time with children can only occur in the context of quantity time.

When our children were younger, I read a book by family physician Richard Swenson, M.D. In *Margin: Restoring Emotional, Physical, Financial, and Time Reserves to Overloaded Lives,* Dr. Swenson explains how families are being destroyed by parents (dads in particular) who leave no margin in their schedule for their kids—and the terrible effects not only on the relationship between parent and child but also on the child's health.

After I had read the book and pondered its truths through much reflection and prayer, I approached my partner in our practice about the possibility of devoting one afternoon each week for each of my children. My typical schedule consisted of morning rounds at the hospital followed by patient appointments in the office for six hours a day (from 9:00 A.M. to noon and from 2:00 P.M. to 5:00 P.M.)—a schedule that left little margin to spend time with my children—just Dad and Kate, or just Dad and Scott.

My medical partner, John Hartman, M.D., and I developed a new arrangement: I would see patients from 8:00 A.M. to 2:00 P.M. on Tuesdays and Thursdays. On those days I'd be able to be home by 3:00 P.M. to meet one or the other of our children at the bus stop (Tuesday afternoons and evenings were for Kate—and for her alone; Thursdays were for Scott). We'd do homework together. We'd take long walks and have long talks about anything and everything. We'd ride bikes. We'd go fishing. We'd go get a milkshake.

I had a blast. An absolute ball. I got to know and love my kids in ways that never could have happened any other way. I learned firsthand that quality time occurs *only* in the midst of quantity time.

In 1998, Kate (by then twenty years old) and I attended a conference for physicians and their spouses. I had been asked to introduce Dr. Richard Swenson. I asked Kate to introduce him instead. She said something like this: "Ladies and gentlemen, when I was a little girl, my daddy read a book that Dr. Swenson had written. The book was called *Margin*. In that book, my daddy learned that if he wanted me to be as healthy as I could be, then he would have to spend some time with me—a lot of time. He would need to create margin in his schedule and in his world for me. So my daddy took time away from work and spent every Tuesday afternoon and evening with me. He has never given me a more wonderful gift. I'll never forget the memories I have from those days."

She turned to Dr. Swenson and said, "Dr. Swenson, I want to thank you for teaching my daddy. Because of what he did, I will never be the same."

She then turned back to the audience. "Dr. Swenson is teaching today about parenting. I encourage you to listen, as my daddy did, so that you can change the life of your kids the way my daddy changed mine."

Then Kate sat down. I'm not ashamed to tell you that both Dick Swenson and I had tears in our eyes.

Parents, hear this loud and clear: Highly healthy kids depend on their relationships with their mom and their dad. Loving parents who give their kids love *and* time give them a greatly increased shot at becoming highly healthy. If your own parents did not give you this gift, then you have a chance to break the cycle with your kids. Oh, and if your kids are grown, perhaps you can influence the relationship your kids have with your grandkids. It's worth the effort!

Better Returns Than the Stock Market

Invest both quantity and quality time in relating to your immediate family—your spouse and children. Devise a specific plan to enhance your parent-child bond and stick to it no matter what the cost. If your kids are grown, consider the potential health benefits to their lifelong well-being of feeling deeply valued and practically supported by you—their parent. It's never too late to provide healing love to your children or spouse.

THE POWER OF A HEALTHY MARRIAGE

Another example of the impact on health of avoiding loneliness and cultivating warm and supportive relationships is found in the research of people who are happily married. They not only tend to live longer than those who are unmarried but also appear to live more highly healthy lives; they have increased quantity and quality of life. I've repeatedly seen convincing scientific and anecdotal evidence that the labor we invest into making our marriages a success will reap significant health benefits for us and for our spouses.

Researchers at Case Western Reserve University in Cleveland, Ohio, published a study of nearly 10,000 married men who had no history of chest pain. Men with elevated risk factors for heart disease, such as high cholesterol, high blood pressure, diabetes, older age, or abnormalities on their EKG were over twenty times more likely to develop angina (chest pain) over the five years of the study. However, those who answered yes to the question, "Does your wife show you her love?" had significantly less angina. Men with the same risk factors who answered no had twice as much angina. The researchers drew this conclusion: "The wife's love and support is an important balancing factor which apparently reduces the risk of angina pectoris even in the presence of high risk factors."

Another study looked at 8,500 men with no history of duodenal ulcers. Men who reported a low level of love and support from their wives had twice as many ulcers as men who felt their wives both loved and supported them.

Those who reported that their wives did not love them had three times as many ulcers as the men who felt their wives loved them.

The companionship, love, and support provided by marriage is associated with lower mortality for almost every major cause of death, at least when married people are compared with the single, separated, divorced, or widowed. Married people are not only more likely to live longer, but they are also more satisfied with living and seem to better survive a variety of diseases. One study showed that the percentage of cancer survivors was significantly higher for the married, as compared with the unmarried, in almost every category of gender, age, or stage of disease. Another study showed that married couples are three times as likely to survive five years after a heart attack than are the unmarried.

After looking at data on more than 12,000 adults, two researchers in England speculated that a spouse could reduce a man's stress and encourage a healthy lifestyle. Yet there may be other factors at play, too. "Exactly how marriage works its magic remains mysterious," they wrote in their report. "Perhaps a strong personal relationship improves mental health and helps the individual to ward off physical illness. More research here is certainly needed."

However, it should come as no surprise to learn that unhealthy marriages are *unhealthy.* Married couples who constantly argue are not nearly as healthy as those who have learned communication techniques that reduce or eliminate perpetual bickering. In one study of couples married an average of forty-two years, those who constantly argued had significantly weaker immune systems than did couples who engaged in fewer disagreements. A study of newlyweds showed that those who exhibited the most negative or hostile behaviors during a thirty-minute discussion of marital problems had measurably reduced immune system function as well as increased blood pressure.

Does this lead me to conclude, then, that if you're in an unhealthy marriage you should divorce? Not at all. In fact, medical studies show that in most cases the long-term effects of divorce can be unhealthy not only for the couple but especially for the children. Many people think that someone who's in a bad marriage has two choices: stay married and miserable, or get a divorce and become happier. But in 2002, the first scholarly study ever to test that assumption was published. The findings were astonishing. The researchers found no evidence that unhappily married adults who divorced were typically any happier than unhappily married people who stayed married. Even more dramatically, the researchers also found that two-thirds of unhappily married spouses who stayed married reported that five years later their marriages were happy. Most surprising of all, the most unhappy marriages reported the most dramatic turnarounds: Among those who rated their marriages as very unhappy, almost eight out of ten who avoided divorce were happily married five years later.

My prescription for an unhealthy marriage is not to amputate a mate but to heal the marriage. It takes mutual effort and steadfast commitment, but it is well worth it.

Measure Your Marital Satisfaction

If you enjoy a healthy marriage—rejoice! As you potentially add years to each other's life spans and lower each other's risk of disease, set aside time to consider specific ways you can enhance your relationship even more. Never take a healthy marriage for granted, but devise a plan for making your spouse feel even more supported and cherished.

If your marriage shows signs of disease, leap into action immediately! Take responsibility to do your part in healing your marriage through improving your communication skills, resolving anger and resentment, and seeking both personal and professional help to give your marriage a chance to thrive.

THE BLESSING OF COMMUNITY

Suppose your family life has not been healthy—or suppose it is not currently healthy. How can you overcome this potential deficit? Research done in Sweden may give you some hope. In a study of the health benefits of social support, Swedish scientists have found that there are two aspects to such support. The first has to do with the primary relationships within your most intimate network—your nuclear family. But the second aspect of social support has to do with how integrated you are with those outside your family—a network that includes your friends, neighbors, and coworkers, or any nurturing support group.

While the close emotional ties within a family play a crucial role in the formation of your identity, self-esteem, and ability to trust others, close personal relationships with colleagues, neighbors, friends, and church or support group members may also play a role in becoming and staying highly healthy. Consequently, you can give yourself the gift of strong relationships with others now and in the future. How I wish Ginny, the lonely widow I mentioned earlier in this chapter, would fill that prescription!

After looking at dozens and dozens of studies, I'm amazed to see the incredible difference that caring relationships can make in someone's health.

Actions as simple as talking with a friend (especially carefully *listening* to a friend), serving in your community, loving your parents, sharing your feelings openly, giving time or money to someone in need, and opening your heart to others can contribute directly to becoming a highly healthy person. Social support, as the term is used in the medical literature, seems in its essence to be *taking the actions* that lead another person to believe that he or she is cared for and loved, respected and esteemed, and linked in as a valuable member of a network (family, church, neighborhood, club, and so forth).

A nearly thirty-year study done in Alameda, California, found that people with less social support (fewer community social ties, no memberships in community organizations or clubs, little or no church attendance) were more likely to die of heart disease or other major illnesses such as stroke or cancer. The researchers could not explain the results by fingering other known risk factors or physical conditions. They could only conclude that a highly healthy person is much more likely to be well connected to other people.

Cardiologists at Columbia University found that people with coronary disease who lived alone were twice as likely to die of a heart attack or to suffer another heart attack. Researchers at Duke University Medical Center found that one-half of heart attack victims who survived their first heart attack and who were socially isolated (defined as those either living alone or saying they had no one they could confide in) were dead within five years. However, in the group of heart attack survivors who were socially connected (either living with their spouse or having someone in whom they could confide), only 17 percent died in the first five years.

More than forty years ago, it was learned that the highest rates of tuberculosis (TB) occurred in individuals with little or no social support—regardless of the patient's economic status. Recent studies at Carnegie-Mellon University and the University of Pittsburgh examined healthy volunteers who were purposefully infected with the virus that causes the common cold. Before infecting their subjects, researchers asked each volunteer about their social relationships and the number of people they spoke to (by phone or in person) at least every two weeks. As the number of social relationships increased, the risk of developing symptoms from the virus decreased. Those reporting only one to three relationships had a fourfold risk of developing a cold compared with those reporting six or more relationships. In short, social support increases a person's resistance to the common cold!

Other studies have found that the majority of supportive and positive nonfamily relationships older Americans enjoy occur among persons they meet at church. A study on church attendance and mental outlook, published in 1987, was based on a random-sample telephone survey of 2,872 people age fifty-five and older who were living in the state of Washington. Among men, religious attendance was significantly and positively related to greater morale after the researchers controlled for ten other variables. In this study, increased church attendance was related to decreased loneliness in men and women. The study indicated that reduced religious attendance increased loneliness by decreasing the number of friends and involvement in social functions.

It is interesting to note, however, that the benefits of religious faith (discussed at length in the next chapter) are much more apparent in those who worship together when compared to those who live or worship in isolation. For example, according to the *Handbook of Religion and Health*, those whose religious activity is limited to listening to radio or watching television appear to be less highly healthy than those who seek social relationships through a faith community. The research reviewed in the book shows that most people are healthier in an active community—a social group of some sort. The author of the New Testament letter to the Hebrews attests to the importance of spiritual community as he writes of spiritual support and worship: "Let us not give up meeting together, as some are in the habit of doing, but let us encourage one another." Obviously, there is now a great deal of medical evidence to support this ancient Hebrew wisdom!

So whether it's church or synagogue, a bridge club, a service club like Rotary or Kiwanis, an exercise group, a book club, or a Twelve-Step support group, the relationships you experience in these social groups and the opportunity they afford you to give and serve will increase the likelihood of your becoming and staying highly healthy.

Cultivate Relationships Like a Garden

Reach out! Don't wait for your phone or doorbell to ring. It is your responsibility—and privilege—to involve yourself in others' lives. Start by making a list of your friends—not casual acquaintances, but people who really know and love you and with whom you interact on a weekly basis. If your list is short, begin another list of things *you* can do to be a better friend. I recommend that my patients check in *every single day*, at least by telephone, with someone close to them. Think of your relationships as a garden that needs to be watered daily—and then do it!

If you're not involved in a social or support group, pick one in your community (you may have to do some research), and *show up*. Even if you're not a "group kind of person," you're more likely to be highly healthy if you feel integrated and useful in your community. Go for it!

"MAN'S—OR WOMAN'S—BEST FRIEND"

For many years I cared for patients at nursing homes. I loved the afternoons I would spend with them. I made sure to touch them and to give them a hug. I tried to brighten their day with a funny story and some shared laughter. We usually prayed together. More often than not, I'd bring one of my children with me. The patients loved seeing the kids and talking to them. For most of my patients, our visit seemed to be one of the highlights of their week.

One day my son, Scott, and I went to see Rosie. She always looked happy to see us. We pulled our chairs next to her wheelchair.

"It's so good to see you!" she exclaimed.

She tousled Scott's crew cut and shouted (she was hard-of-hearing), "What's up, Skinny?" (her favorite term for his lean six-year-old frame).

"It's good to see you, too, Rosie. What's up with you?" I inquired.

She looked around and then leaned toward us. "Boys," she whispered, with a mischievous smile on her face, "I've got a new love in my life—a new man, don't ya know. And boy oh boy, does he ever make me feel young!"

As I was running through the likely nursing home candidates in my mind, I watched Rosie tilt her head back. She inserted two fingers between her lips and unleashed a whistle that could have awakened the dead.

"Here, Rusty!"

We could hear the clicking of his toenails as he galloped down the hall and into Rosie's room. The large golden retriever leaped onto the arm of her wheelchair, knocking it back a bit. As he licked Rosie's face, she laughed and laughed.

Rusty transformed that nursing home. He improved Rosie's overall health. And he changed my view of pets in health care facilities.

A few years ago, Barb and I were touring a nursing home on the campus of Truman East Medical Center in Kansas City, Missouri. A good friend, Paul Williams, M.D., was displaying his accomplishments. Being a former country doctor, Paul instinctively knew the value of animals and the positive health effects they can have. His nursing home was not only sparkling clean, staffed by caring personnel, and filled with sunlight, it was also "staffed" by two cats, one dog, and a flock of finches in a beautiful flight cage. To watch the residents and staff interact with the animals was a pleasure. Who owned whom was not a question easily answered. But everyone—staff, patients, and pets—seemed highly healthy, or at least highly happy!

A number of medical studies have shown that people who have pets are healthier than those who do not—even when all other factors are the same. In one cardiac study, only 1.1 percent of those who owned dogs died during the study, compared to 6.7 percent of those who did not have a pet. In another study, which followed patients for one year after discharge from a hospital after a heart attack, 6 percent of pet owners died in that year compared to 28 percent of those who did not own pets. In yet another study, Medicaid recipients who owned pets made fewer visits to the doctor or the hospital than those who did not have pets.

To my delight, there's a whole new branch of medicine called *pet therapy*. Trained owners and their pets volunteer to visit the sick and shut-ins—at home or in health care facilities. It's one more way to help people become more highly healthy.

Pampered Pets Pamper Health

If you already enjoy the company of a pet, then you've already filled a prescription for increasing your health and happiness. If you don't have a pet, don't wait for a pet therapy expert to bring one to you in a nursing home someday! If you have the time, ability, and the home arrangements to care for a pet, consider going to the Humane Society and picking out a dog or kitten to care for and love. If you don't want to own a pet, follow my friend Cynthia's example and volunteer at an animal shelter on weekends. The big smile I see on her face every time she talks about her work at the shelter leads me to believe that her weekly "dose" of puppy love is making her more highly healthy.

GET CONNECTED!

The bottom line of dozens of studies from around the world is simply this: Healthy relationships matter. Remember, loneliness can kill. Are you avoiding it like the plague? If not, are you willing to step out and pick one or more of the prescriptions I've recommended and apply it to your life? Or are you thinking, *Can any of this make a difference?* Great question. Researchers have an answer.

Psychologists at McGill University took a group of heart attack survivors who were being discharged from the hospital and assigned them to one of two groups. Both groups received the best heart care from the cardiologists and their family physicians. However, one group (the intervention group) also received a monthly phone call from the researchers. If the researchers sensed any psychosocial problem, a specially trained nurse was dispatched to the patient's home. Just this simple relationship enhancement resulted in a 50 percent reduction in the patients' death rate after one year. Providing just one support person who called once a month but who was available to help if any help was needed—just *one* caring, helping person—contributed to longer lives for the patients studied.

Here's the sad part: Had a pill obtained this same result, that pill would be making millions of dollars for its manufacturer and *every* heart attack patient would be demanding that his or her insurance company pay for the pill. Yet this research—with its amazing conclusion—is virtually unknown. Imagine the potential impact if every church or synagogue provided this kind of caring service for its worshipers! Can you imagine the results if hospitals routinely provided this service for the patients they discharge?

In another study, Stanford researchers randomly assigned women with metastatic breast cancer to receive usual care or usual care plus a weekly support group designed to help the women manage stress and improve relationships. Guess what? The support group patients lived *twice* as long! At UCLA, patients with malignant melanoma who participated in only six ninety-minute sessions with a support group that also provided relationship training had a 50 percent reduction in death and recurrence when compared with the usual-care patients. Over the six years of this study, more than three times as many patients in the nonintervention group died as compared to the group that received support.

Listening—*really* listening—also improves your health. Researchers at the University of Maryland have shown that when a person listens, his or her blood pressure lowers significantly. However, if the "listening" person is instead thinking about what he or she is going to say next, then the blood pressure does not go down.

Finally, *giving* support to others will improve your health. In one study of more than 700 elderly adults, the more love and support they offered to others, the more their own health improved. For relationships to be highly healthy, there must be reciprocity—a mutual decision to give and receive love and support. People who are only on the receiving end and never give back are much less likely to be healthy.

Some social science researchers today talk more about networks and connectedness than about social support—recognizing that, in the long run, relationships are reciprocal. It's not always what you're getting but what you're *giving* that counts—especially as people age. What often keeps older people going is recognizing that they have something profoundly valuable to give.

One of the first things I prescribe for patients who suffer both from poor health and from loneliness is that they become active in volunteer work. I always kept a list of volunteer and mission opportunities my patients could choose from. I insisted that they commit to this activity. Almost invariably, when they filled this prescription—when they began to give of themselves— the change in their countenance and in their disease process was dramatic.

When Alice moved to our small town and chose me as her family physician, her medical problem list was extensive. But as I got to know her, I was most concerned about her loneliness. I talked to her about the many opportunities in our community for her to use her talents and skill. She refused to try even one thing.

Then came a decisive office visit. I gave her the bad news at the very beginning. "Alice, I have to ask you to find another physician."

She just stared at me with an expression somewhere between pain and shock. "You've got to be kidding. Are you leaving town like my other doctor did?"

"No, ma'am," I replied, "I'm not leaving town. But I still have to ask you to find another doctor."

"Are you firing me?"

"Yep. I'm firing you."

"For what!?"

"For not getting involved. Alice, the plain truth is that loneliness is killing you. You need to volunteer to help others, not because they need you, but because *you* need them. Your giving to them will improve your health. Unless you're willing to start helping others—this week—I'm giving you the pink slip."

"Are you blackmailing me?"

"No, I'm caring for you—because I really do care about you. And if you want me to keep providing medical care for you, then you need to follow this suggestion and begin to care for someone else. If you're not willing to start this week, I'll help you find another doctor."

"Humph." Alice dropped her head. "Hmmm . . ."

The silence dragged on.

"My boys are telling me I need to get out. Pastor is telling me I need to get out. Now you're telling me to get out of your office if I don't get out."

I waited through another moment of silence.

"Well, it's just so hard starting over with a new doctor that I guess I'll have to give this fool idea of yours a try. Where should I start?"

I gave her a list, and we discussed the options. A vocational center near her home seemed to pique her interest—a place where persons with mental impairments received job training and employment.

Three weeks later, I received a call from the center's director. "Best thang ever happened to us down here is ol' Alice," he told me. "Her laughter shakes the rafters. She's one big ball of energy—here the minute we open, and I near 'bout got to kick her out in the evening. She done shook this place up. Kids love her. Staff loves her. I love her. Thanks for sending her, Doc."

Two weeks later she was back in my office for a checkup. "Alice, your blood pressure is better, your pulse is slower, your blood sugar is better, you've lost a bit of weight, and you look better. What's going on? What are you doing to improve so much?"

"Aw, Doc, I guess I'm exercising a bit—like you've told me. I'm eating a bit better; that's probably making a difference. But it's *not* that fool thing you *made* me do—going down to volunteer at the center. I mean, it's not *too* bad going down there—but I don't think that's why I'm better. I'm just doing it to keep from having to change to another doctor."

I smiled at her. I think she smiled back. When I left my practice in Kissimmee, Florida, Alice was still at the center and practically running it. And she was more highly healthy than she'd ever imagined she could be.

WHAT IS YOUR RELATIONSHIP IQ?

Are your relationship habits ones that would predict a high degree of health? Or are your relationship skills likely to negatively affect your health? Drs. Virginia and Redford Williams of Duke University developed a rather extensive questionnaire that became one of my favorite ways to measure this with my patients. I first met the Williamses when they were guests on my television show right after they had written the book *Lifeskills*. I was already a fan after reading their excellent book *Anger Kills* and using its principles in my practice.

Their Relationships Questionnaire is based on several standardized instruments, including the Interpersonal Support Evaluation List (developed by Carnegie-Mellon psychologist Sheldon Cohen) and the CES-D scale (developed by the Center for Epidemiological Studies of the National Institute of Mental Health). The Williamses also credit the work of Ilene Siegler and Robert Karasek in developing this questionnaire.

It's easy to take, and it's available in appendix 1 with the permission of the Williamses and their publisher. Give yourself thirty minutes or so for the test. Read each question slowly and carefully, and circle "T" for "true" and "F" for "false." If both answers seem likely, just choose the one that seems more likely to be correct. Remember, you should choose the one most likely to reflect your true feelings. Avoid choosing an answer that reflects how you think you *should* feel or act. (If you don't want to make marks in this book, just take a piece of paper, number from 1 to 114, and write your answer by each number. The scoring key is at the end of the questionnaire.)

What should you do if your score is abnormal on any portion of the questionnaire? First, remember that these are just *screening* tests. They do not diagnose anything. No self-screening test is 100 percent accurate. But it can provide useful information for anyone who potentially has a problem. If your test score is abnormal, see someone who can help you sort out what the results may *really* mean for you. It doesn't matter if it's your family physician, a pastoral professional or counselor, or a psychiatrist or psychologist. Get some help. Call today.

Scrutinize, Score, and Study Your Relationship Wheel

Spend several hours studying your results on The Relationships Questionnaire. Consider journaling about what you've discovered about yourself and your relationships. Most important, *discuss* the results—and any concerns you might have—with someone whose wise counsel and kind heart you trust. It could be a close friend, a member of the clergy, or a counselor. See what kinds of solutions you can come up with—*together.*

Avoiding loneliness and pursuing healthy relationships can increase the likelihood of your becoming a highly healthy person. Concentrate on and improve the relationships you already have. The fact is that by improving your relationships you can increase the health of others you care about. As you build communication skills, as you treat others with compassion and respect, as you display grace and commitment, your kindness toward them and your relationship with them will help them improve their health. It's almost like an infectious disease. When you spread grace to others and they "catch" it, they will be more likely to spread it to others.

The absence of loneliness, the fostering of socialization and positive relationships, and the development of constructive and graceful communication styles can increase not only the likelihood that you will be highly healthy but that those around you will be healthy as well.

I hope you've learned that if you are angry or hostile, you can drive people away and increase your personal loneliness. If you are cynical or depressed, you'll be inclined to withdraw from others and increase your personal loneliness. If you have uncaring relationships or refuse to socialize with others, you may suffer dire health consequences.

If any of this is true for you, I assure you that there is hope. To continue on the journey to becoming a highly healthy person, fill some of this chapter's prescriptions for building stronger and healthier relationships. As you do, you will, in turn, avoid loneliness like the life-threatening plague it is.

CHAPTER EIGHT

Cultivate a True Spirituality

The Essential of Spiritual Well-Being

I met Jerry, a physician, at a medical conference where I gave a presentation on how the latest medical research continued to support what I'd been witnessing in my own practice for years, namely, that a person's *spiritual well-being* has a significant positive impact on his or her physical, emotional, and relational health.

Jerry asked me to join him for lunch one day, and I was fascinated by his comments on spirituality. It quickly became apparent that Jerry and I were talking about two very different things!

"I don't mean to dispute anything you reported on the findings regarding spirituality and health, Walt," he said, "but I must tell you I just haven't seen those kinds of results in my own practice. Like you, I take an inventory of sorts with many of my patients, especially those who have chronic health problems. I encourage them to go to church, volunteer at a local charity, join a Rotary club or community service group. Some do, but I can't say I've seen them become much healthier or happier. In fact, one patient's been a longtime member of one of the oldest churches in town, but he came to see me six months ago, complaining of disabling insomnia and depression. I prescribed the appropriate medications, but he doesn't really seem to be getting better. I'd like to believe that his spiritual activities could improve his situation, but I'm not seeing the evidence. What do you think?"

I told him about Fran, a patient who was a decade-long inspiration to me before she died at the age of ninety-two. Fran attended church regularly and volunteered to help others in her community whenever she could (she'd been doing both for more than seventy-five years!). She was a woman of deep personal faith. She rarely visited my office more than once or twice a year, but when she did she always made some reference to her love for God and commitment to her spiritual journey.

During our last visit she said, "I know I'm not going to live forever, but who would want to? I feel pretty good right now, but I'll be jumping for joy when I meet my Maker face-to-face!" Her face literally glowed. "For twice as long as you've been alive, I've been enjoying his companionship and thanking him for his faithfulness in helping me be who I think he wants me to be. I talk to God all the time, and I'm here to tell you—he listens! It's been a good life, walking hand in hand with him and other folks who know him like I do."

Jerry looked perplexed. "Wow! I've never heard *my* patient say anything like that. In fact, one of his frustrations is how pressured he feels by all his commitments at church; I think he's a deacon or something. Frankly, he sounds pretty miserable, even though he's plenty dutiful. Maybe I'll try to delve a little deeper the next time I see him—you know, see what his religion really means to him. I know he could use some of the joy and peace your patient enjoyed for so many years."

This physician clearly had made the connection between the kind of spirituality I was talking about and how it affects a person's overall well-being. There is a difference between true spirituality and an external religion in which people go through the motions of religious duties but lack any personal relationship with God. I hope this church member eventually discovered a personal and meaningful relationship with God and became more highly healthy.

WHAT KIND OF SPIRITUALITY DO YOU HAVE?

Before we reflect further on true spirituality, it is important for you to consider your philosophy of life. Most of us make one of two basic assumptions: Either we (1) view the universe as an accident and our existence on this planet a matter of chance, or we (2) assume some divine intelligence beyond space and time that not only gives the universe design and order but also gives meaning and purpose to life. How we live our lives, how we approach the end of our lives, what we perceive, how we interpret what we perceive, how we approach wellness and illness and suffering—all these things are formed and influenced consciously or subconsciously by one of these two basic assumptions. If you consider these two views as polar opposites—two ends of a spectrum, if you would—then it's easy to imagine many points, philosophies, or beliefs between the two endpoints.

On one side are those who believe that human beings are the products of chance, existing for a short time in an impersonal cosmos, determining our own fate or having our own fate determined for us. The belief is that "the right stuff"—right marriage, right job, right kids, right amount of money, right car or house or clothes—will bring joy, peace, and satisfaction, and that increasingly sophisticated technology will provide cures and answers to the world's most desperate problems.

On the other side are those who believe that human beings were individually created and formed by a personal and loving Creator who is omnipotent, omnipresent, and omniscient (those are big words for all-powerful, present in all places in all times, and possessing all knowledge). The textbook for this view—the Bible—maintains that we can choose to trust our Creator and live according to the purpose he designed for each of us, or we can rely instead on our own finite plans and efforts. We have a choice.

The Bible also promises that if we choose to allow our Creator to fill and empower our very souls, then we will develop spiritual fruit that endures, regardless of our circumstances or the state of our physical, emotional, or relational health. There is no doubt that technology has potential to provide cures and answers to some of our most desperate problems—but *not* for our most basic problems. And all those "good things in life"—right marriage, right job, right kids, right amount of money, right car or house or clothes—can only be *added to* the most important element of wellness, namely, seeking, knowing, and pleasing our Creator. If we believe in and trust God, if we make an intimate relationship with him a priority, if he controls and empowers our lives and we seek our purpose in his grand design, then we will experience wholeness at the deepest level of our being.

Augustine, a fourth-century theologian, put it this way in what is perhaps his best-known statement: "You have made us for yourself, O God, and our hearts are restless until they find rest in you." And Episcopal Bishop Edmund Lee Browning asks, "What does it take to be happy?" Here's his answer: "I think we are happiest when we know ourselves to be in the service of God, focused on a reality larger than ourselves. This is true even when that service is hard, which it often is. No amount of inconvenience or effort can take that joy from us; it is why we are here."

Take a Microscope to Your Beliefs

Take a few minutes to consider these two points of view on the origins of the world—and any in between. One end of the spectrum assumes that there is no God. The middle of the spectrum (the religious view) believes that God wants to have a relationship with us, but that we must earn or deserve this relationship. Many of the world's religious, and even many Christians, see themselves and their world through this lens.

The other end of the spectrum believes that God wants to have a personal relationship with people and that there is nothing we can do to deserve or earn his favor and love. Because of the wrong decisions we have each made, we fall short of God's measure that would allow us to know him personally. That's the bad news. But the good news is this: God made a personal relationship possible for each of us by sending his Son, Jesus, to live a perfect, exemplary life and to sacrifice his life to pay the price for all our wrongdoing. According to this view, all we have to do is accept his love. He doesn't force us, however. We are free to choose.

In your journal replicate the illustration below. Place an *X* where you'd locate your beliefs as of today. Take your time; consider how you *really think and live*—not just what you've been taught through the years—and be honest about how you view yourself, God, and life. Then ask yourself where you want to be on this scale in the future. Place an *O* on the scale to represent this desire. Put today's date by the scale.

I have no	My relationship	I have a highly
relationship	with God is	meaningful
with God	distant or	personal relation-
	formal	ship with God

FAITH THAT WORKS

There are many definitions of spirituality, some of which include elements that strike me as unhealthy. Because there are a number of definitions for related words (such as faith, morality, and religion), for the purposes of this book I'll always be referring to *true spirituality* when I talk about the spiritual health wheel.

True spirituality is distinguished from the broader terms (faith, morality, or religion) in that it involves an ever-evolving, authentic, and personal relationship with God that is not bound by race, ethnicity, economic status, or class. This relationship promotes the wellness and welfare of others and of self. It includes the beliefs and values by which an individual lives; it results in the visible spiritual fruit of love, joy, peace, patience, kindness, goodness, faithfulness, gentleness, and self-control. The concept is clearly outlined in the Bible and is often referred to by Christian theologians as *true spirituality*.

Researchers have shown that those who internalize biblical teachings—who frequently pray, apply what the Bible says to their lives, believe they have a close relationship with God, and practice what they preach—have high levels of satisfaction in life, a sense of well-being, and overall happiness. True spirituality is also more likely to be associated with a wide variety of positive physical and emotional health outcomes.

Research indicates that these benefits are not as significant when one just goes through the motions of religious tradition. People who merely attend worship services and programs in their religious community tend to experience an external faith that is less likely to be associated with positive physical or mental health outcomes. Researchers since the 1960s tell us that some people use religion in a self-serving, utilitarian way. "Persons with this orientation," they say, "may find religion useful in a variety of ways—to provide security and solace, sociability and distraction, status and self-justification. The embraced creed is lightly held or else selectively shaped to fit more primary needs. In theological terms the extrinsic type turns to God, but without turning away from self."

Religion, for them, according to Dr. Dale Matthews, professor at Georgetown University School of Medicine, "is a means to obtaining another end—health, security, status, power—even though they may not be consciously aware of their own ulterior motives." In his book *The Faith Factor,* Matthews says that those who use their religion for their own purposes (using a paraphrase and inversion of John F. Kennedy's words) "ask not what they can do for their religion, but what their religion can do for them."

As you can imagine, persons who rate higher on the "true spirituality" scales (compared to those relying on "external religion") are more likely to experience mental and physical health benefits—significant benefits, in fact. For example, recovery from a major depression has been shown to occur much more rapidly and completely for those with the highest ratings of true spirituality. A lowering of blood pressure, better surgical outcomes, less substance abuse, and longer survival have also been noted in the research.

According to researcher George Barna, men and women with a true spirituality say they are most satisfied with their present life (91 percent)—an upbeat frame of mind that may be related to the fact that they are the least likely to say they are lonely (8 percent), in serious debt (9 percent), or stressed out (16 percent). The percentage who admit to high levels of stress was less than half the level measured among adults connected with (extrinsic) faiths (33 percent) or those who said they were atheistic or agnostic (42 percent).

This 2002 Barna survey, of over three thousand randomly chosen adults in the United States, found that "although they are slightly less than 8 percent of the American adult population, atheists and agnostics possess self-perceptions that clearly stand out from those of citizens who maintain some definable faith preference. The nonfaith segment placed highest among the five niches in claiming to be stressed out (42 percent), concerned about the future (68 percent), and lonely (14 percent). They were the least likely to be satisfied with their life (68 percent) and to be concerned about America's moral state (60 percent)."

It would only be fair to mention that in some studies there is no correlation between spiritual health and physical or mental health—and in some cases there is a negative effect. However, these represent a small minority of the total studies, and most of these studies have significant limitations. Some have been poorly designed, while others used only the most superficial measure of religious activity—asking perfunctory questions such as, "Do you attend church?" In spite of this, it seems clear that those who rarely attend religious services or those who have shallow personal faith are at higher risk of experiencing illness.

Certain religious beliefs and activities can adversely affect both mental and physical health. Some forms of faith, spirituality, and religion can be restraining rather than liberating and life enhancing. Sadly, religion has sometimes been used to justify hypocrisy, self-righteousness, hatred, murder, torture, and prejudice. An external religiosity that separates people from community and family, that encourages blind devotion and obedience to a single charismatic leader, or that promotes religion or spiritual traditions as a healing practice to the total exclusion of research-based medical care is likely, over time, to adversely affect health—and may even *prevent* you from becoming a highly healthy person.

A true spirituality can assist you in acknowledging your limitations without causing you to despair of your circumstances. Research has shown that when people become ill, most rely heavily on spiritual beliefs and practices to relieve stress, retain a sense of control, and maintain hope and a sense of meaning and purpose in life.

For example, one study of elderly patients undergoing elective cardiac surgery showed that lack of strength and comfort from religion was independently related to the risk of death during the six-month period following surgery. Another study of elderly poor forced to move from their homes showed that those who were more religiously committed were twice as likely to survive the two-year study period as persons without such religious commitment. The most influential study variable was the strength and comfort derived from religion.

The first two heart attack patients I cared for during my first year in private medical practice had opposite views on religion. Our forty-bed hospital in Bryson City, North Carolina, was simple, but we provided excellent care. We had a four-bed intensive care unit, and it was into this unit that I admitted two men, each of whom had suffered his first heart attack.

These guys were a lot alike. They had loving and devoted spouses and families. They were only a year apart in age and had similar medical histories—except Bob was a smoker and Earle was not. Both had been relatively fit and healthy prior to their heart attacks. If I had to draw their physical, emotional, and relational wheels, they'd look very much alike.

However, their spiritual wheels were significantly different. Bob was a man of deep and abiding faith who exuded an inner peace. He seemed optimistic about "what the Lord is going to teach me through all this." During morning rounds, I'd find him reading his Bible—and he'd excitedly share what God was teaching him that day. Both his wife and his pastor spoke of how Bob "walked his talk." When I made evening rounds, I'd meet people at his bedside— friends, neighbors, and colleagues—who would testify that they had come to know God in a personal way because of Bob's testimony and the life he lived.

Earle, on the other hand, was very negative. "Doc," he'd scowl, "I just can't understand why God would do this to me!" He seemed angry at God— and he'd take his anger out on the staff. And yet, Earle was *more* "religious" than Bob, if you measure religion only in external terms. Earle attended his church on Sunday mornings, Sunday evenings, and Wednesday evenings, and he "went visitin' on Tuesdays." He didn't miss a revival meeting or church activity. He was a deacon and a Sunday school teacher. But his family cowered when he shouted at them, and the hospital staff tried to avoid him as much as possible.

Their EKGs and the blood levels of their cardiac enzymes revealed that Earle and Bob had suffered similar heart attacks in terms of location and size. The two men's clinical courses, however, were anything but similar. Bob's recovery was uncomplicated, and he left the hospital on the fifth day after admission. Earle experienced a much stormier course. He had a worsening of his heart damage and several scary episodes of a dangerous abnormal heart rhythm. When he left the hospital twelve days after admission, his heart was scarred for life. He never recovered physically or emotionally. He died at home of a massive heart attack less than a month later.

As I reflect on these two patients, I think it's fair to say that Bob had a high level of true spirituality. Earle, on the other hand, practiced a negative and external religion. When folks came to visit, he'd put on his pious face, but when they left, his old nasty self would reappear.

Hear me, now. I'm *not* saying that a personal relationship with God is an insurance policy—a guarantee—against disease. It is not. But the medical research is clear that the deeper your true spiritual faith, the more likely you are to have a better mental and physical health outcome. You are much more likely to cope well with illness and to recover from disease. Earle was my first patient to show me that what the research suggests is true.

Evaluate Your Spirituality – What Type Are You?

Do you consider your personal faith to be an expression of true spirituality, or an expression of an external religion? Are you as consistent as you'd like to be in living out your faith in your daily life? Why or why not? Now consider one or more things you can do, beginning today, to transform your faith to become an expression of a stronger true spirituality. Spend some time recording your thoughts in your journal or on a piece of paper.

Don't give in to the temptation to skip this test. If you don't honestly evaluate your spiritual wheel, you won't be able to improve its inflation and balance.

WHAT SCIENCE SAYS ABOUT SPIRITUALITY

If spiritual health is crucial to becoming and staying highly healthy, then we should be able to find proof in the medical literature—and there is plenty!

In his book *The Relaxation Response*, Dr. Herbert Benson of Harvard Medical School discussed the many studies showing that spiritual disciplines such as prayer and meditation can reduce the stress response (elevated blood pressure, heart rate, and breathing rate). A national adult study in 1991 by sociologist Christopher Ellison found that the frequency with which people both prayed and attended religious services had a significant impact on their health status, regardless of their age. The more involved people were in religion or religious activity, the better their physical, emotional, and social health measures. (Ellison also published a national study in 1989 showing that both frequency of religious attendance and devotional intensity were associated with increased levels of life satisfaction.)

The *Handbook of Religion and Health* examines the religion and health relationship by documenting more than 1,600 research studies and medical review articles that have explored the relationship between religious or spiritual activity and emotional, social, and physical health outcomes. The vast majority of these studies demonstrated that a patient's religious and spiritual beliefs can be clinically beneficial and play an important role in both coping with and recovering from illness. Here are just a few of the many positive findings:

Longer Life

Between 1987 and 1995, a nationwide study of more than 21,000 adults showed a seven-year longer life expectancy in those who attended religious services more than once a week when compared to those who never attended.

Lower Blood Pressure

A study of 401 men in Georgia, published by Duke researchers in 1989, showed lower blood pressure (and less hypertension) in those who considered religion very important *and* who attended church regularly.

Improved Surgical Outcomes

In 1995, Dartmouth researchers published a study revealing that patients to whom faith was important were three times more likely to be alive six months after open-heart surgery than patients for whom faith was of no importance.

Shorter Hospital Stays

In a 1998 study, Duke researchers showed that people who attended church weekly were not only less likely to be hospitalized than those who did not attend church regularly, but when they were admitted, they had a shorter length of stay.

Improved Mental Health

According to a 1997 Duke University study of more than 4,000 adults age sixty and older, frequent attendees at worship services had significantly reduced rates of depression and anxiety.

Overall Well-Being

Epidemiologist Jeff Levin's 1994 research showed that adults age sixty and older who considered themselves religious had fewer health problems and rated their overall functioning higher than those who considered themselves nonreligious. The authors of the *Handbook of Religion and Health* draw this conclusion: "Persons with high religious involvement are less likely to abuse alcohol and drugs; experience less hypertension, heart disease, stroke, cancer, and disability; and live longer. Better physical health invariably translates into a higher level of well-being, given the strong association between physical and mental health."

WHAT GINGER CAN TEACH US ABOUT THE SPIRITUAL WHEEL

Ginger was a perfect example of the kind of impact positive spirituality or religiosity can have on mental and physical health. When I met her, she had no room in her life for spirituality. I saw her for a myriad of chronic physical, emotional, and relational problems. With counsel and medications we were able to muddle through over the years. Ginger didn't get worse, but she never got better.

When I asked about her spiritual history, I discovered that, though she had grown up in church, she viewed church people as hypocrites. As soon as she could leave home and church, she did. She struggled through three marriages—each one more abusive than the last. She wrestled with chronic depression, panic attacks, and anxiety. She lived with constant back pain. The effects of alcohol and tobacco had scarred her liver and lungs. Her relationships at work were often strained. In short, she was a mess.

Throughout the years, I encouraged her to pay special attention to her flat spiritual wheel. She would laugh and comment that the other three weren't much better. "But," I'd assure her, "I think they could be—*would* be—if you'd ever turn some of your attention to God."

She'd always smile. "Dr. Larimore, please don't ever give up on me. But for now, I'm just not interested in spiritual things."

Everything changed when I delivered her first grandchild. Children, particularly babies, have a way of turning a family's heart toward home—and toward God. Ginger, who was there when the baby was born, joined in my prayer of thanks for a safe pregnancy and birth. It was Ginger who encouraged her son and daughter-in-law to get back to church now that they were parents. And she began to witness a life-changing spirituality in them. She saw their marriage improve and her son's chronic battles with irritable bowel syndrome virtually disappear. Ginger's heart slowly began to soften toward spiritual things.

One day, as her office visit drew to an end, she *asked* me to pray for her—after ten years of refusing to allow me to pray for her at the end of our time together! It was a major step in her spiritual journey. I did pray for her that day. And then I asked if she'd be willing for me to check her level of spirituality.

"Is there a blood test for that?" she asked.

I chuckled. "No, but you could answer a brief questionnaire that would help us both. How about it?"

She agreed.

The best possible score was a one, which showed very high levels of true spirituality. Unfortunately, but not surprisingly, Ginger scored near the bottom.

"What do I need to do?" she asked, in a tone that reminded me of a small child.

"Well," I advised, "I think a consultation would be in order."

She looked shocked. "A *consultation?* With who?"

I smiled. "Ginger, over the years we've put together a spiritual consult team made up of men and women who have a strong personal relationship with God. They love helping other people find their own spiritual path."

"Do they charge?" she inquired, and then quickly added, "Does my insurance cover this type of care?"

"Unfortunately, most insurance companies don't cover spiritual care," I said. "But these folks delight in doing this type of care. There's no charge."

I arranged for a woman about Ginger's age to begin spending time with her. Ginger began to change—slowly at first, then more and more quickly. What was most remarkable to me, my partners, and my staff was this: As Ginger began a personal relationship with God—as she became active in a church, as she began to pray and to study the Bible, to reach out and volunteer in her community—she discovered a new ability to cope with and overcome many of the problems she had in her other three health wheels.

Ginger was learning that the spiritual wheel really is the key—the most important of the wheels, the one connected to the "power drive."

THE "EVIDENCE" DISCUSSED IN THE MEDIA TODAY

Doctors and scientists aren't the only ones fascinated by the role of faith in physical and emotional healing. During the last decade it's become increasingly common to read in lay publications about the connection.

For example, the May 2001 issue of *Reader's Digest* ran an article titled "Why Doctors Now Believe Faith Heals: Because They're Finding the Medical Evidence." *U.S. News & World Report* noted that nearly two-thirds of the nation's 125 medical schools now include course work on spirituality issues. Back in 1993, only three schools had similar offerings! *The Atlantic Monthly*, a popular read among the intellectual establishment, highlighted the results of a study suggesting that intercessory prayer can aid in another person's recovery.

Numerous respected newspapers across the country have also reported the healing power of religious faith and prayer. In late 2001, *The Seattle Times* printed the results of a thirty-year study of 2,600 people, showing that those who attended weekly services led healthier lives and had better overall health habits than those who were less likely to attend church.

The belief that prayer and faith can play a major role in personal health is also catching the eye of large medical organizations. A recent article in the *Milwaukee Journal Sentinel* told of how the Joint Commission on Accreditation of Healthcare Organizations—a widely respected entity—now provides questions and guidelines for a spiritual assessment of all patients entering hospitals or outpatient medical facilities.

According to an article in the *Los Angeles Times,* the late Dr. David Larson, past president of National Institute for Healthcare Research in Rockville, Maryland, noted that there is a growing file of evidence that most people who are ill would welcome some care of the soul along with treatment for their physical illness. Suggesting that religious beliefs and a supportive faith community can assist with strengthening a patient's coping mechanisms, Larson asserted that prayer and religious faith are as important as conventional medicine. I think he's right.

Television reporters have noticed the research, too. CBS's *The Early Show* and ABC's *Good Morning America* both featured segments in 2001 on the benefits of prayer and a personal faith. On CBS, Dr. Harold Koenig reaffirmed studies that "religious people" tend to live an average of seven years longer than those who don't identify with a personal faith.

This groundswell of media interest attests to the fact that people are interested in and value what the research shows about a neglected factor of clinical care, namely, spiritual assessment and support.

However, having pointed all this out, I must encourage you to exercise wisdom when reading about such research. Why? Well, just because something is related to good health does not guarantee that everyone doing it will be healthy. Or just because something is related to bad health does not guarantee that everyone doing it will be unhealthy.

Millie is a good example of the latter. Most people are aware that tobacco use is a major risk factor for cancer. The use of tobacco products is associated with a reduction in both the quality and quantity of life. Smokers, for example, are far more likely than nonsmokers to get lung cancer and heart disease. Their lives are usually less healthy and shorter than the lives of nonsmokers. Not so for Millie, though. She was ninety-four years of age when I left Bryson City. Most days you could still find her sitting in her rocking chair on the front porch. If she wasn't smoking her corncob pipe, she was dipping snuff. She was still going strong—and kept going until she died at the age of ninety-nine.

On the other side of the coin was Claudia. At ten years of age, she was a deeply religious person—a genuinely good person. She was active in her faith, yet she was struck down by leukemia before her eleventh birthday. Claudia was one of the exceptions. According to a lot of medical research, when large groups of people are examined over time, deep and personal religious commitments are almost always associated with highly healthy people who generally live longer, healthier lives.

ASSESSING YOUR SPIRITUAL HEALTH WHEEL

How does your own spiritual wheel look? Full of air and bouncing along in proper balance and alignment? Or a little flat? Maybe you haven't maintained it for a long time and it's taken a beating from the nails you've picked up along the road of life. Or maybe when you've taken a careful look at your own health "car," you've realized you have only three wheels—the spiritual wheel is completely missing!

Spiritual distress or crisis occurs when people cannot find meaning, hope, joy, satisfaction, love, peace, comfort, strength, and connection in life or when conflict occurs between their beliefs and what is happening in their life. Medical studies are fairly clear that this distress can have a negative and damaging effect on physical, mental, and relational health.

I'm convinced that God wants us to be as physically and emotionally healthy as possible. He wants us to enjoy healthy relationships with others. But most of all, he wants us to have a healthy relationship with him. The best way I know to become a highly healthy person is to develop a true spirituality that can result in the most important and enduring form of health and vitality.

Do you need a road map for the journey? For starters, I recommend the simple self-test below, developed by George Barna. The questions are designed to help you determine how well you are doing in your personal spiritual journey. Based on Barna's two decades of research on people's spiritual development and fulfillment, these questions focus on the key factors involved in spiritual health. While no evaluation tool can perfectly assess every dimension of your spiritual life, your responses can give insight into how you are doing spiritually. Be honest. The value of this inventory is to help you identify strengths and weaknesses, which can then lead you to a more focused and meaningful spiritual journey.

BARNA SPIRITUAL JOURNEY ASSESSMENT

Developed and provided by George Barna, Barna Research Group, Ltd., Ventura, California

How true is this characteristic of you?

1 = Not at all or never	4 = Often or usually
2 = Not much or rarely	5 = Completely or always
3 = Somewhat or occasionally	

1. You maintain an intense level of respect, awe, humility, and gratitude toward God—in acknowledgment of his superiority and perfection. _____

2. You effectively share the substance of your faith with people who have an interest in it. _____

3. You pray for the needs and future of others. _____

4. The choices and decisions you make are based on spiritual principles and values. _____

5. Your speech and behavior pleases God. _____

6. When you pray, you both speak and listen to God. _____

7. Worship is not just an event you attend—you try to live your life as an act of worship to God. _____

8. You are held morally and spiritually accountable by others who know and care for you. _____

9. You give away your time, abilities, and money sacrificially for the benefit of the needy. _____

10. You fight injustice and inequality. _____

11. You strive to live out the "Golden Rule"—to love other people as you want them to love you. _____

12. Your attitudes, values, and thoughts please God. _____

Add up your score. A score of 48 or higher indicates you are likely to be spiritually healthy; a score of 24 or lower indicates you may not be spiritually healthy at present. Record your score in your journal, so you'll be able to compare your current score with future scores.

Evaluate Your Barna Score

Does your score on the Barna questionnaire surprise you? If your score is lower than you might expect or want it to be, look for two or three things you could do, beginning today, to raise your spiritual health quotient.

If you can't think of anything to do, is there a pastoral counselor who might be able to counsel you in this area? If so, call him or her today and make an appointment to have a chat. He or she would be delighted to provide counsel and guidance.

Simple self-tests such as the Barna one are merely the first level of checking your spiritual wheel. I highly recommend a detailed spiritual assessment for Christians developed by Pastor Randy Frazee and his staff at Pantego Bible Church in Fort Worth, Texas. The Christian Life Profile (CLP) has been used by church consultants and church leaders around the globe and, according to Frazee, is optimally used in the context of biblical community or in a small group of Christians.

Pastor Frazee has graciously worked with me to adapt his comprehensive questionnaire to make it available to you in a much simpler form. We're calling this adaptation the Spiritual Life Profile (SLP). Its approach derives from Luke 10:27, where Jesus notes that the two essentials of spiritual vitality are to love God and to love your neighbor as yourself. Using these two essentials of spiritual health, this self-assessment tool produces a profile of your spiritual life from the biblical perspective.

The questions measuring your love for God provide a detailed way to look at the vertical spoke of your spiritual wheel; those measuring your love for neighbor give a more detailed measure of the horizontal spoke. Measuring these spokes will help you assess where you are compared to what I consider to be the ideal profile—the one lived out by Jesus.

The SLP is designed to help you discover both the strongest areas of your spiritual life and the areas where there are the largest gaps in your spiritual life. You may already have a preliminary sense of your spiritual wheel, based on the "spoke exercise" in chapter 2 (see pages 46–48). But the tools in this chapter enable you to take a more comprehensive look at this wheel—perhaps from different angles and with a stronger magnifying glass.

Investing the time to honestly answer the SLP questions will help you target specific areas in your spiritual life that you'd like to develop. Now it's time for you to go to work again. You'll find the SLP in appendix 2.

Take the Spiritual Life Profile

Be sure to set aside an hour or so to work on the Spiritual Life Profile tool. It is *not* an assessment to take quickly. As you answer each question, ask yourself, "How can I improve or grow in this area?" Remember: be honest. Don't fill out the questionnaire the way you think you *should* be—or the way others think you should be. Indicate instead where you have been spiritually over the past few months. Where you were last year or ten years ago isn't relevant to what you may need to do *now* to increase the health of your spiritual wheel.

The SLP is divided into a set of ten core beliefs and practices and ten core virtues. Ten of these allow you to assess your love for God, and ten assess your love for neighbor. The SLP first measures how you love God by measuring three beliefs (for example, a personal God, compassion, and stewardship) and seven practices (for example, how much you give of your time, treasure, and talents). Then the tool measures how you love your neighbor by measuring ten virtues or spiritual fruits (for example, love, joy, and peace). It allows you to compare yourself against the model set forth by the Bible—but without endorsing any particular denominational belief or doctrine.

Review the Spiritual Life Profile Once a Day

For the next few weeks, spend time each day studying your results from the Spiritual Life Profile. Consider journaling about what you're discovering about yourself and your relationship with God and with a faith community. Most important, *discuss* the results with someone whose wise counsel and kind heart you trust. Talk over any concerns with a close friend, a member of the clergy, or a faith-based counselor. See what kinds of solutions you can come up with together to "round out" your spiritual wheel.

Once you've completed the evaluation, I suspect you'll identify some deficiencies. This is *not* the time to get discouraged. Let me reassure you: The first step to becoming highly healthy is to honestly identify those areas in which you sense there is a need for improvement.

Think of an abscess, which continues to fester until finally you become aware of it and go to a doctor to have it lanced—to release the collection of pus. Yes, lancing may create discomfort, but unless or until the infection is released—until the bad stuff is drained—the tissues cannot and will not become healthy. Until you know which areas need treatment, you can't improve your spiritual health.

Perseverance Pays Off

Unless you're a superhero, you may be feeling a bit discouraged—and that's perfectly normal. But don't quit. Your health and your family's health depend on your perseverance.

No one said this journey would be easy. And before you know it, you'll be further along the way to becoming a highly healthy person.

For those areas of the spiritual wheel in which you sense a need to grow, find someone you respect or admire spiritually to discuss strategies for becoming more highly healthy. Pick up the phone and call your pastor (if you don't have one, find a Bible-believing church and call the church office) to set up an appointment to review your spiritual wheel assessments. Talk about the strategies you can utilize to inflate your spiritual wheel. Or call Focus on the Family (1-800-A-FAMILY) and ask about resources that can guide you. Remember, perseverance pays!

True spirituality is the path to spiritual wholeness. For most of us it is a lifelong pursuit. A healthy spiritual wheel is the foundation to the hope, health, and well-being for which we all long. How can we settle for anything less?

CHAPTER NINE

See Yourself as Your Creator Sees You

The Essential of a Positive Self-Image

She was, without a doubt, the saddest patient I had ever cared for.

Suzie had a beautiful smile and a pleasant laugh that, when she was well, would pour forth in peals. She was a devoted high school teacher. Her students loved her. The ones I talked to felt blessed to have her as their teacher. Her colleagues seemed to respect and admire her. The principal of the small private school where she taught raved about her. "One of the best teachers I've ever supervised!" he exclaimed.

Her morbid obesity did not seem to be a detriment to her social relationships. But even in her mid-twenties, Suzie was struggling with diabetes and severe asthma. She had difficulty staying on the strict diet that diabetics must follow, and she adamantly refused to exercise.

Her most troublesome medical problem was her asthma. In the first few years I cared for her, she had four to six hospital admissions per year for severe asthma attacks. She ended up on every medication possible, yet still had frequent asthma attacks. Visits to several pulmonary and allergy specialists weren't helpful.

Suzie claimed that her spiritual faith was important to her and maintained that she regularly attended worship services and was active in her church. Yet whenever we had time to chat at her office visits, she'd often confess that she saw herself as pitiful and pathetic, as possessing no self-worth and not being worthy of love or respect. Perhaps because of her negative self-image, Suzie didn't care about dressing nicely, and she rarely wore makeup. I asked her once if her lack of makeup was for religious reasons.

"No," she sighed forlornly, "I just don't see the purpose."

I looked carefully for the source of this terrible self-image. Was there suppressed anger? Child abuse? Sexual abuse? Overly strict parents? Was there any addiction to pornography or drugs? Chronic depression? She adamantly denied all of these.

Finally Suzie agreed to see a psychologist.

The psychologist called after a few visits. "Walt, I've never really met anyone like Suzie. She has the worst self-image of anyone I've ever worked with. This is going to be one tough case." And in the end the psychologist couldn't help Suzie.

Through the years, Suzie saw several pastoral counselors and other therapists. None could make a breakthrough. She went on spiritual retreats—to no avail.

She and I would pray together during her office visits. She seemed to be working hard to manage her diseases, but her asthma and diabetes steadily worsened. She worsened. And, at the age of thirty-one, she died.

When her death certificate came, I wanted to write as the cause of death *Rotten self-image*—and as the secondary cause of death *She hated herself.* But instead I wrote, "Respiratory failure secondary to asthma, diabetic ketoacidosis and sepsis—aggravated by morbid obesity and cardiomyopathy." But all of these diseases had, in fact, been made worse (if not caused) by her poor self-image—her hatred of herself.

Based on her physical and emotional symptoms, I'm convinced that Suzie had been severely abused as a child. Whoever abused her—physically, sexually, emotionally, spiritually, or maybe even in all four ways—no doubt convinced her that great harm—maybe even death—would come to her, should she ever reveal these events. Perhaps she had buried it so far into her subconscious that it was no longer accessible to her rational mind. But no matter the cause, the effect of Suzie's self-hatred was obvious—and fatal.

Through the years, I've cared for scores of patients who suffer from a poor self-image. Although most don't die from this malady, most are diseased from it. In fact, they often suffer terribly—physically, mentally, relationally, and spiritually. In their book *Happiness Is a Choice,* psychiatrists Paul Meier and Frank Minirth write, "We believe there are three primary sources of emotional pain. One of these primary sources is *lack of self-worth* (a low self-concept)."

The Bible has a lot to say about our self-esteem as well, making it plain that our capacity to love God and to love others (the two greatest commandments) is directly related to the way we view and treat ourselves.

A teacher of the Jewish religion once asked, "Of all the commandments, which is the most important?"

"The most important one," answered Jesus, "is this: 'Hear, O Israel, the Lord our God, the Lord is one. Love the Lord your God with all your heart and with all your soul and with all your mind and with all your strength.' The second is this: 'Love your neighbor as yourself.' There is no commandment greater than these."

This teaching underscores what I see as the three most basic spiritual and emotional needs of all people:

1. a positive relationship with God
2. a positive relationship with oneself
3. positive relationships with others

If a person has no love for himself, then how can he love his neighbor as himself? And how can a person love herself in a healthy way unless she is bolstered by the love of God? Knowing how God sees us is key to building positive self-esteem and to loving God and others out of full and secure hearts.

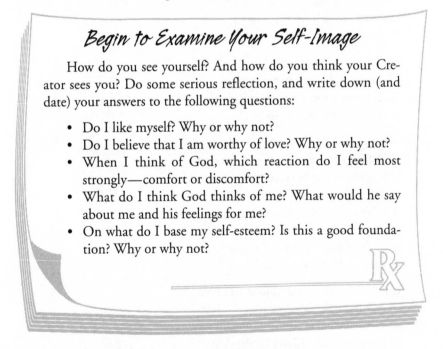

Begin to Examine Your Self-Image

How do you see yourself? And how do you think your Creator sees you? Do some serious reflection, and write down (and date) your answers to the following questions:

- Do I like myself? Why or why not?
- Do I believe that I am worthy of love? Why or why not?
- When I think of God, which reaction do I feel most strongly—comfort or discomfort?
- What do I think God thinks of me? What would he say about me and his feelings for me?
- On what do I base my self-esteem? Is this a good foundation? Why or why not?

ONE OF A KIND—FOR A PURPOSE

Noted personality theorist Alfred Adler is said to have coined the term *inferiority complex.* An inferiority complex can cause or be caused by a poor self-image. Yet everyone I've ever treated who suffers from an inferiority complex has one thing in common: Their inferiority is the result of comparing themselves to others—a not only inappropriate but highly unhealthy thing to do.

Why? According to the Bible, we are designed by our Creator *not* to be like other people—not to be like any other person ever born! No other person in history is like us. No other person has had or ever will have the same set of genes or the same fingerprints or brain waves or the exact same life experience and perspective.

David, one of the kings of ancient Israel, eloquently described God's hand in our design :

> O LORD, you have searched me
>   and you know me.
> You know when I sit and when I rise;
>   you perceive my thoughts from afar.
> You discern my going out and my lying down;
>   you are familiar with all my ways.
> Before a word is on my tongue
>   you know it completely, O LORD.
>
> You hem me in—behind and before;
>   you have laid your hand upon me.
> Such knowledge is too wonderful for me,
>   too lofty for me to attain.
>
> Where can I go from your Spirit?
>   Where can I flee from your presence?
> If I go up to the heavens, you are there;
>   if I make my bed in the depths, you are there.
> If I rise on the wings of the dawn,
>   if I settle on the far side of the sea,
> even there your hand will guide me,
>   your right hand will hold me fast.
>
> If I say, "Surely the darkness will hide me
>   and the light become night around me,"
> even the darkness will not be dark to you;
>   the night will shine like the day,
>   for darkness is as light to you.
>
> For you created my inmost being;
>   you knit me together in my mother's womb.

I praise you because I am fearfully and wonderfully made;
    your works are wonderful,
    I know that full well.
My frame was not hidden from you
    when I was made in the secret place.
When I was woven together in the depths of the earth,
    your eyes saw my unformed body.
All the days ordained for me
    were written in your book
    before one of them came to be.

How precious to me are your thoughts, O God!
    How vast is the sum of them!
Were I to count them,
    they would outnumber the grains of sand.
When I awake,
    I am still with you.

Our human nature is to compare ourselves to others. And this will almost always result in feelings of inferiority. In my opinion, one of the most beautiful and classiest women of the last century was Princess Diana (or "Di" as she was called by her hordes of admirers). Apparently much of the English-speaking world shared this assessment. Yet there was one person who did not—the princess herself. She reportedly was stricken with an awful case of poor self-esteem.

My guess is that Princess Diana, like any of us who make the mistake of comparing ourselves to others, believed a lie—that somehow we are less worthwhile if we are not "like" or "better than" the people we admire or the ones we think "deserve" approval and love from others and from God.

Teenagers are especially vulnerable to and affected by this "compare and despair" problem. Who among us, as we think of our teenage years, didn't feel different or awkward or weird? Virtually all teenagers feel inferior—especially if they aren't aware of how God made them and sees them in all their glorious uniqueness. Rather than appreciating their uniqueness and celebrating how special they are in God's eyes, they believe that they need to conform—that not being like everyone else is a problem they need to solve. This pressure is so great in childhood and adolescence that those who dare to be authentic and different are often ostracized, bullied, ridiculed, or forsaken.

Psychiatrists Frank Minirth and Paul Meier wrote a book called *The Healthy Christian Life* in which they use the acronym A-C-T-I-O-N to describe some of the common ways that teenagers handle their feelings of inferiority. See if you recognize your own tendencies in this list—even if you're "all grown up"!

- **A = Alike-ism.** "I can hide myself by being like everyone else. I must not be different in appearance and behavior."
- **C = Compensation.** "I'll find what I can do well and concentrate on it, whether it's sports or good grades or whatever. That way I will be accepted and respected for something."
- **T = Trip out.** "It's impossible to make the pain go away, so I will hide in drugs and alcohol."
- **I = Introversion.** "If I am a quiet little mouse, maybe no one will know I exist. If I open my mouth or take some initiative, I might make a mistake and people would laugh at me. I can't take the risk."
- **O = Obstinate.** "I will pretend that I am tough and crude. I can bluff people into thinking I am confident by the way I show disrespect to others and treat them like trash."
- **N = Nitwitty.** "I will be a clown. I will do stupid things and make people laugh, especially at me. When they laugh, I won't let myself feel that they are laughing at me for any reason other than because I make them laugh. I feel important when people are happy because of me."

Take ACTION by Looking at Yourself

Do you see the teenager in you in any of these traits? Consider each one, and think of a time in the past year when you have demonstrated any of these coping mechanisms. Did you use one because you felt inferior to someone else? Why did you feel that way? To the extent that you can recognize these tendencies in yourself and begin to overcome them, you will make progress toward becoming a highly healthy person.

HOW TO PUMP UP A DEFLATED SELF-IMAGE

You may be thinking, *I hear what you're saying, but I'm just not sure it's true. I don't feel God's love. I don't feel his acceptance. I don't feel unique or special. I don't feel like he sees me—at all!*

Well, I remind you that solid convictions should *never* start with feelings. Never! In fact, *faith is not a feeling.* Belief starts with making a choice—a conscious act of the will, a decision. You see, your feelings—your emotions—will always be changing. However, facts don't change (the Bible's timeless and unchanging truths, for example). If you choose to place your faith in feelings, then you're going to be in trouble because your feelings are always subject to change—and thus your faith will, too.

Your faith will only be as solid as the thing you place your faith in. It's not just the act of believing but *what you believe in* that will determine your degree of health. For example, if you place a great amount of faith in the thin ice on a pond—believing that it will hold your weight as you walk on it—then no matter the amount or quality of your faith, you're still going to get wet and cold. On the other hand, even a little bit of faith placed in a *thick* sheet of ice will be rewarded. You'll be able to cross over safely. If you're willing to place your faith in what God says about who you are and what you mean to him, then the positive emotions—and the higher degrees of health that accompany them—will follow.

So if your self-esteem is low, what can you choose to do to increase the likelihood of becoming highly healthy? Throughout the years, I've developed an advice sheet (a prescription of sorts), to help my patients who suffer from a poor self-image. All eight items are supported both in the Bible and by scientific research.

1. Place Your Relationship with God at the Center of Your Life

There is significant scientific evidence that our faith in God is associated with a large number of positive mental and physical health outcomes.

The week I was writing this chapter, I received an e-mail message from a young woman who had been cared for in our medical practice for several years. She wrestled with a number of emotional and relational problems that overflowed into physical distress. She was a classic neurotic at the age of fifteen!

For the years that I'd been her doctor, I tried to encourage her to develop some sort of spiritual life—to pay attention to her spiritual health wheel and come up with a strategy to inflate and balance it. She hadn't been open to these suggestions. She left for college and I didn't see or hear from her until this message arrived:

> *Dear Dr. Walt, I need to catch you up with me. First of all, I want you to know that I've never been better. I've never felt better. I'm following your advice on nutrition, exercise, and sleep—and no doubt that has made a tremendous difference. In fact, I remember you kidding me that my diet was a "nutritional den of iniquity." Well, things are better in that department!*

The most difficult part of your advice to follow was to try to begin a personal relationship with God. I guess I never felt that he would want to know me. I certainly never felt that I was anything special to him.

Here at the university, I have run into some really neat girls in my dorm. They claimed that they knew God personally—that he had changed their lives. One of them told me that God loved me—that he had made me just the way I am. That he wanted to have a relationship with me. That he wanted to give me joy and peace. That he had a special plan just for me.

Well, Dr. Walt, I know you've told me some of that. But, I guess I just wasn't ready to hear it—or accept it—until now. This year I've begun that personal relationship with God. And putting him at the center of my life has put everything in balance. I feel like a new me!

What an encouraging update to read! I hope it suggests to you a way in which you can become healthier as well. I believe that the underlying truth of our lives is that we were created by a loving God—in the very image of this God—and that knowing him, serving him, pleasing him, and worshiping him will fulfill our primary purpose in life and eternity. In short, we are hardwired to please and to glorify him in all we think, say, and do.

Reflect on Your Creation

The first step in seeing yourself as your Creator sees you is to understand his view of who you are. Take a moment to reflect on the fact that he formed you in the womb, that he knows you and desires to have a personal relationship with you. How does this make you feel? Better already, I hope!

- Make a list of your talents and how you are using them. Are there ways you could use them more effectively?
- Make a list of how you are using your treasure. Are there ways you could be a better steward of your monies?
- Make a list of the ways you effectively use time; then list the ways you think you might be wasting time. What can you do this week to make better use of your time?

Begin today to thank God for who you are and for the many gifts he's given you. This attitude of gratitude opens the door to learn even more about how he sees you.

2. Read, Memorize, and Meditate on Bible Passages Daily

For years I've been giving my patients an assignment to memorize and meditate on portions of the Bible that are relevant to a health issue with which they are wrestling. Several studies have shown that people who spend time reading and reflecting on the Bible daily have better health outcomes. One researcher examined the relationship between Bible study and a healthy marriage. He found that 59 percent of those who read the Bible regularly and applied it to their marriage challenges reported high levels of marital health. The researcher concluded, "There was a fairly strong relationship between both prayer and Bible reading and marital adjustment," and, "A strong commitment to religious practice and ideals can enhance marital stability."

Other studies have found that daily Bible reading was associated with greater life-satisfaction in the lives of both physicians and their patients and greater degrees of hopefulness. Bible reading also may be associated with a protection against alcoholism and depressive symptoms.

Betsy had been living with dysthymia—a form of chronic mild depression—for some time. Both her sister and her mother had the same problem, and all three were being treated with appropriate antidepressant medication. Betsy came in one day complaining that her depression was much worse.

We spent some time discussing several recent life events that might have played a role in her growing depression. We discussed changing her antidepressant medication, making changes in her diet, and possibly adding dietary supplements that have alleviated depression in some patients. I spoke of some of the medical studies that suggest how getting enough exposure to light and increasing her amount of exercise could decrease her symptoms. Last but not least, I asked if she'd be willing to memorize and meditate on a Bible passage I'd found to be helpful for folks wrestling with depression. She seemed interested. So I wrote a prescription: "Memorize Psalm 1 and meditate on it for 15 minutes twice a day." I also gave her samples (and a prescription for) an antidepressant medication that might work better for her.

I saw Betsy in the office about a month later. When I walked into the exam room, the "normal" Betsy greeted me. Her eyes fairly sparkled.

"Wow!" I exclaimed. "You sure look good. That new medicine must have really helped."

"You mean this one?" she asked as she handed me the unused samples and the unfilled prescription.

"You didn't try the new medicine?"

"Nope. I just stayed on the old one. But the prescription that helped me the most was to memorize that psalm." Then she proceeded to quote the entire psalm—word for word!

"Doctor," she said, "that was one of the most helpful things I've ever done. I got so much from that Scripture. Are there others I should memorize?"

I was delighted to write out a prescription for several additional Bible passages I'd found helpful for lifting the spirits and enhancing self-worth.

A number of amazing things happen to people who commit to the discipline of reading the Bible and memorizing portions to reflect on during times of meditation. One of the most astonishing things that can happen is that one's whole way of thinking can be renewed and refurbished. In fact, the Bible tells us: "Do not conform any longer to the pattern of this world, but be transformed by the renewing of your mind." A poor self-image can be transformed into positive self-esteem as we discover how much God really loves us and how passionately he wants our lives to be full and meaningful.

Many of my patients who suffer from poor self-esteem were programmed that way (just like a computer is programmed) when they were young. Perhaps this programming was carried out by overbearing or neglectful parents or by cruel siblings or classmates. This kind of negative programming invariably results in faulty thinking. It can make us believe we are bad. It distorts the way we see ourselves and can keep us from experiencing God's love and receiving his grace. It can cause us to worry and to be filled with self-doubt, self-criticism, and self-condemnation. It can cause us to doubt that there is a God, much less believe that he loves us. It can cause us to be suspicious of the motives of others and to doubt their care or love for us. Bottom line, wrong thinking, or wrong "self-talk," can keep us from becoming highly healthy.

We have no control over any of the past programming of our brain. Yet the good news is this: No matter what the cause of the initial programming— and the fact that this past input will almost always have an effect on how we feel, think, and act—we can learn new ways of thinking and behaving. Our Creator designed us that way!

The "renewing" of our minds is usually a gradual process, and it can be enhanced by reading, memorizing, and meditating on the Bible. King David compared a highly healthy person to a tree growing by a river:

> Blessed is the man
>> who does not walk in the counsel of the wicked
> or stand in the way of sinners
>> or sit in the seat of mockers.
> But his delight is in the law of the LORD,
>> and on his law he meditates day and night.
> He is like a tree planted by streams of water,
>> which yields its fruit in season
> and whose leaf does not wither.
>> Whatever he does prospers.

Find Encouragement in the Bible

Many Bibles include a list of verses to read and meditate on for particular problems or issues. If you visit a Christian bookstore, the sales associates can help you pick a Bible that meets your needs.

For example, the *NIV Encouragement Bible* includes inserts that list Bible verses that answer many of the fundamental questions every human being has at one time or another. Here are just a few:

> *Why do I sometimes feel distant from God?*
> *How can I grow in my love for God?*
> *Who can possibly understand the depth of my sorrow?*
> *Does God see my pain and hear my cries for help?*
> *How can my struggles be used by God to help others?*
> *How do I deal with anxiety? Fear? Anger? Loneliness? Depression?*
> *How do I deal with despair? Bitterness? Pain?*

You can also find books that cover specific subjects and cite Bible verses that help in these areas. For example, Dr. Billy Graham's daughter, Anne Graham Lotz, has reissued Samuel Bagster's classic *Daily Light* and included some of her favorite verses that share biblical wisdom on specific concerns.

3. Spend Time in Meditation and Prayer Daily

Prayer and times of solitude are high priorities in the lives of highly healthy people. Prayer is simply conversing with God. Meditation is purposefully concentrating and listening with our spiritual ears to what God has already said in Scripture and what his Spirit communicates to our spirits during conversation.

For me, this spiritual conversation begins as soon as I wake up each morning—and so I need to set the alarm clock for at least a half hour before I have to begin my day's duties. When I wake up, God is the first thing in my thoughts. Before I even get out of bed, I thank him for my night's rest and for the gift of the new day in front of me. I pray specifically that in all I do in the day that lies ahead I'll grow to know him more deeply and honor him more completely.

Several medical studies discuss the effects of prayer—both on those who pray daily and on those who are prayed for. One study showed a positive correlation between religious activity such as prayer and Bible reading and satisfaction in life.

Researchers believe that time spent in meditation and prayer—especially when joined with Bible study—takes a person's focus away from a potentially pathological concentration on self—a focus that not only lowers self-esteem but also reduces life-satisfaction and well-being. By concentrating on ourselves and our problems, while failing to see the "bigger picture" related to any suffering we are experiencing, we can actually contribute to our own demise.

Investing as little as five to ten minutes a day in meditation and prayer can begin to change you.

Take Time for Yourself

Here's a stunning fact: Most men and women invest very little time in themselves. But those who do take time each morning for prayer and meditation—whether it is with Bible and a cup of coffee in hand at the kitchen table, or outside taking a short walk—invariably report that they feel better prepared for the day.

Medical studies show that small breaks scattered throughout the workday can increase your energy, your productivity, and your satisfaction. Those who invest in a ten-minute power nap each afternoon tend to perform better at work.

If you've never considered investing time in yourself, now is the time to start. Set your alarm clock fifteen minutes earlier. Get out of bed and enjoy the luxury of time alone—for you and your Creator.

4. Avoid Negative Self-Talk

Being overly critical of ourselves—regularly beating ourselves up—makes a low self-esteem worse every time. People can improve their moods, their attitudes, and their overall health by changing the way they think and the things they tell themselves about themselves, life, and God. What we think is what we declare to ourselves in the privacy of our own minds. What *is* the power in positive thinking?

One large review concluded that, while an optimistic attitude does wonders for patients' recovery, negative attitudes and critical self-talk decrease one's likelihood of becoming highly healthy. Researchers reviewed sixteen studies (spanning thirty years) that focused specifically on patients' attitudes after surgery. Across a wide range of clinical conditions, from lower back pain to heart surgery, patients who felt they would do well in recovery did do well. Patients whose attitudes were negative or who talked negatively about the surgery— they were scared or pessimistic about their recovery—did not recover as quickly or as fully as the optimists did.

The apostle Paul wrote, "Whatever is true, whatever is noble, whatever is right, whatever is pure, whatever is lovely, whatever is admirable—if anything is excellent or praiseworthy—think about such things. Whatever you have learned or received or heard from me, or seen in me—put it into practice. And the God of peace will be with you." What we think and how we think— and how we "talk" to ourselves about what we think—has a direct impact on our peace of mind. The type of thinking Paul has in mind improves our moods, our immune functions, and thus our health.

How Full Is Your Glass?

If you have a habit of talking to yourself in a criticizing way, or if you tend to have a pessimistic outlook on life (seeing the glass as half empty instead of half full), then making a decision to see a pastor or a counselor who can help you change your way of thinking could be a highly healthy intervention for you.

You may want to pick up the book *Unbreakable Bonds*, written by psychologist Cheryl Meier and her father, psychiatrist Paul Meier. The Meiers discuss a number of superb strategies for overcoming negative self-talk. (My daughter, Kate, and I had the privilege of writing the foreword for the book.)

5. Build Family Intimacy

Many—perhaps most—of my patients with poor self-esteem have poor family relationships as well. The experience of acceptance and love in a family is more important to health than many people imagine.

If you have a family, you can begin to improve your health by improving the quality of your family life. You know the saying, "It's not the quantity of time you spend with someone, but the quality"? Well, that's utter nonsense. Quality time comes *only* in the context of quantity time. Quality time cannot be preprogrammed or scheduled. It happens only when we are willing to spend adequate amounts of time with the people we love.

For spouses, I recommend a date with your spouse at least once a week. Barb and I started this delightful practice when I began medical school nearly thirty years ago, and we've continued it up to this very day. Nowadays, our weekly date involves going out for breakfast one morning a week when we're not already traveling together on business. We also take one or more romantic weekends together every year. In addition, we seek out weekend conferences every few years to build our marriage skills. Barb and I consider these events and the time we spend together—time focused on each other and on how we can grow personally and build each other up—crucial to our individual health, our self-esteem, our marriage, and our family life. It's *our* time to talk, to listen, to communicate, and to iron out differences.

For parents, determine to spend quantity and quality time with your children *every* day. It might mean making sure you're home for family supper at least four nights a week. It might include reading to small children, taking extra time for bedtime rituals, or planning weekly dates with each child (no matter what their age) so you can listen carefully to whatever is on their hearts.

The day Kate, my oldest child, turned six years old, I was talking to my dad on the phone. "Walt, congratulations!" he said.

"For what?" I asked, just a bit puzzled.

"Well, one-third of your life with Kate is over."

It took a moment to realize what he was telling me. Kate would likely leave our home at the age of eighteen. Indeed, one-third of my up-close-and-personal parenting time was gone. *That's it!* I thought to myself. *I'm not about to let this time slip away.* Then and there I determined to spend more time with my kids—while I still could.

After talking it over with Barb, we made a commitment to have dinner as a family at least five evenings a week—not in front of the television, not at a fast-food restaurant, not even ordering in a pizza, but we would cook a meal *together* and sit down to eat *together.* By choosing to *dine* rather than just feed ourselves and our kids, we made up our minds to be fully present with each other—to eat slowly and talk and laugh and genuinely enjoy each other.

Is this highly healthy? You bet it is! In fact, according to freelance writer Charles Downey, "Families eat less when they dine together because they talk, and that slows the speed of eating, giving the stomach's fullness signals a chance to work. Even small amounts of food start sending satiety signals to the brain in 20 minutes." Children who dine with their parents tend to have healthier diets than those who don't. But that's not the only reason to make family meal-times matter. Experts say that sitting down together is one of the most important activities of family life, where sharing personal news and information should be a priority. Children in this type of environment tend to flourish.

Research published in the *Journal of Epidemiology and Community Health* examined more than 200 youngsters who were living with their parents. The teens in this group who needed mental health services ate a meal with their family at home (on average) less than five times a week. The healthier kids dined with their relatives at least six times a week. The researchers concluded, "Sharing daily meals is a unifying ritual that promotes adolescent mental health."

In 1997, the American Psychological Association published a study that demonstrated the crucial role of the family meal in the lives of teenagers. The study found that the most well-adjusted teens—those with better peer relationships, more academic motivation, and few, if any, problems with drugs and depression—ate dinner with their families at least five evenings a week. Other research by the University of Minnesota and the University of North Carolina showed similar findings: Drug use, sexual behavior, violence, and emotional stress were less likely in households where the parents were present at crucial times, particularly during meals.

Finally, since so much of our self-esteem is related to our parents' (and other close relatives') love for and acceptance of us, it is worth every ounce of effort to try to reconcile with parents and relatives with whom we have poor relationships or unresolved issues. Also, as grown children, we must choose to spend quantity time with our parents, if possible. The Bible says, "Honor your father and your mother, so that you may live long." Spending time with our father and mother is one of the best ways to honor them, and God promises to bless us for that behavior.

Spend Time with Your Spouse and Your Kids

Here's your assignment: Keep a small notebook or pad of paper and a pen by your bedside. Each night for the next two weeks, jot down the number of minutes that you spend alone just talking or listening to your spouse and each child who lives at home—*not* including time watching TV or time in the house together. Only include eye-to-eye time. (You may be stunned at how little time you give to each other.) At the end of two weeks, have a family meeting. Develop strategies to help you spend more time with each other.

6. Spend Time Each Week with Highly Healthy People

The impact of relationships on our becoming highly healthy cannot be understated. Solomon, considered one of the wisest teachers of all time, gave good advice on choosing our friends: "As iron sharpens iron, so one man sharpens another," and "A cheerful heart is good medicine, but a crushed spirit dries up the bones." In other words, choosing good friends can improve our health!

How many friends are enough? Can you have too many? Can you have too few? There is danger in having just one intimate friend. If he or she were to move away or for any other reason leave you, the gaping hole would be hard to fill. But having too many friends isn't always highly healthy either. Solomon wrote, "A man of many companions may come to ruin, but there is a friend who sticks closer than a brother." Frank Minirth and Paul Meier concur: "Intimacy is what is needed . . . not quantity."

Take One Dose of Cheerful Friendship

As you consider these principles—dining with your children, improving your relationship with your parents, and spending more time with highly healthy people—determine which area is the weakest for you. In which area could you make improvements? Then determine at least one thing you can do—and *will* do—to increase your or your family's health in this area.

7. Do the Things That Bring Joy and Satisfaction

Nurturing your God-given hopes and dreams is a must for folks who want to become highly healthy. Why? Because those activities and aspirations bring you true joy and satisfaction. They are the things most likely to bolster your self-esteem.

I find it amazing that unhappy, discontented folks with a poor self-concept continue—day after miserable day—to do those things (often self-destructive or at least nonnurturing activities) that only make them feel worse. They refuse to do those things that are virtually guaranteed to improve their self-image and increase their feelings of satisfaction. They make excuses. The tip-off for me is when they say, "I can't . . . " or "I've tried, but . . . " You fill in the blank. I can only interpret these as excuses—plain and simple.

Whenever I encounter someone who tries to use one of these excuses—to avoid responsibility for their actions—I stop them in midsentence and have them change their "I can't . . . " to "I won't . . . !" In *Happiness Is a Choice*, the authors write, "If an individual changes all his *can'ts* to *won'ts*, he stops avoiding the truth, quits deceiving himself, and starts living in reality."

Harry is a great example. He worked for the family business—delivering bottled water. He made a good living, but it wasn't what he was created to do. He felt an emptiness, a gnawing dissatisfaction. What Harry really enjoyed was growing orchids.

Finally, through a variety of experiences and with the encouragement of his wife, Harry decided to leave the bottled water business and purchase a nursery business in a nearby town. He did the research, checked the references, and negotiated for a transition of ownership—which reduced his risk of failure and allowed the owners to teach him the business.

I met Harry and Ellen after they were established in their new business. They are role models for me—they absolutely *love* what they do, which manifests itself in joy and health.

As an aside, Harry knew a stockbroker named Don who made a ton of money but was miserable. After a few years of helping Harry with the nursery business on Saturdays, Don decided to leave the world of finance and become a nurseryman alongside his friend.

Recently I visited Harry and Don at their nursery in central Florida. It was a sight to behold. Although not the richest men in the world financially, they are among the richest in many other ways—and above all, they are highly healthy!

8. Serve Others

People who have a healthy self-esteem are not self-absorbed. In fact, being comfortable in our own skin empowers us to serve and truly give of ourselves to others—just the way Jesus commanded us to. Loving our neighbors as ourselves is a virtue of the highest order. Yet those who practice this discipline will always testify that "you get more than you give." People who make serving others a high priority have the greatest likelihood of becoming highly healthy.

Steve Wilson, a psychologist and self-proclaimed "joyologist," says, "There is a kind of unhappiness that cannot be repaired by getting because it requires giving. There is a kind of dissatisfaction, disappointment, and absence of joy that is remedied by giving something out, doing something for others. . . . Happiness is an inside job that consists of becoming disillusioned that material acquisition is a measure of your worth, remembering who you really are (precious), finding your source, laughing often, serving with love."

Researchers studied 2,153 older people in Japan and found a fascinating pattern. Self-reported health status among men tended to be higher among those who helped other people—and the more that these men helped others, the better their health. Those who were more involved in helping others (and had a higher degree of health) were also the men who engaged in private religious practices. One possible explanation for this finding is that having strong social ties and a sense of life-satisfaction improves a person's immune function.

Serving a Sense of Satisfaction

Take a few moments to reflect on your life over the last year or two. Do you have feelings of satisfaction as you ponder what your life has been like? Are you involved in helping or serving others? Do you see a link between helping others and your sense of satisfaction?

If you tend to spend most of your time pursuing your own interests and goals, I encourage you to find specific ways you can make serving other people a higher priority. What will you do differently in the month ahead in order to become more highly healthy in this area?

Think about a place in your community or church where you can serve. Commit to serving at a food pantry, a homeless shelter, a hospital, a senior citizen center, the humane society. There are hundreds of other options. Pick one—any one. But choose a place and a time to give of your time and talent to others less fortunate. In one way, your health depends on it.

A LOOK IN THE MIRROR

How is your view of yourself? When you look at yourself in the mirror or think about how you've lived your life, do you feel positive or negative? Do you feel healthy—or unhealthy?

Highly healthy people almost always have a positive view of themselves. I'm *not* saying that they are conceited—or that their egos are overinflated—but that they've come to accept themselves, warts and all, and to respect themselves.

If you suffer from a deflated self-image, it's time to take another look in the mirror. See yourself as God sees you. He designed and created the person you see reflected there. You were designed to have a life that is full, meaningful, and infused with a sense of well-being. God designed you to experience and dispense—every day—love (rather than self-contempt), joy (rather than disappointment), peace (rather than anxiety), patience (rather than petulance), kindness (rather than meanness), goodness (rather than misery), faithfulness (rather than distrust), gentleness (rather than harshness), and self-control (rather than self-absorption).

You will have to invest much time and effort in the prescriptions and advice I've dispensed in this chapter. It's work—hard work! Motivational speaker Jim Rohn wrote, "We must all wage an intense, lifelong battle against the constant downward pull. If we relax, the bugs and weeds of negativity will move into the garden and take away everything of value." As this spiritual fruit grows in your life, you will become more and more stable and whole. The dividends are literally out of this world.

Consider this: By seeing yourself as your Creator sees you and learning to incorporate his plan and design into how you live and what you do, you will become empowered to live out God's purpose for your life. I believe that your Creator has designed you for a very specific purpose—and being true to that purpose will result in genuine and lasting joy and satisfaction.

Our purpose is often reflected in our deepest dreams, desires, and hopes. What are yours? I'll look at this topic in the next chapter.

CHAPTER TEN

Nurture Your Hopes and Dreams

The Essential of Discovering Your Destiny

One of our favorite places in the small hamlet of Bryson City, North Carolina, where I began my medical practice, is the Hemlock Inn on the outskirts of town on a small mountain above Galbreath Creek. This simple and pleasantly rustic inn serves delicious homemade mountain food. Its restaurant is always "standing room only" at breakfast and dinner, where meals are served family style at large round tables from a large lazy Susan in the middle.

Because of the seating plan, guests tend to visit—and when people visit, they invariably seek common ground. "Where are you from?" "What do you do?" "Do you have kids?" "This your first time here?" More often than not, these kinds of questions lead to the discovery of a mutual friend, a similar life event or interest—and the launching pad for an in-depth conversation.

In 1979, when we first visited the Hemlock Inn, Barb and I were nearing thirty years of age—while most of the guests were retirees. The one common thread in just about every person we met was that only then, in the twilight of their lives, were they beginning to live their dreams. Almost to a person they had delayed for decades doing something they longed to be able to do. One was beginning to paint with watercolors. Another was learning to play the hammer dulcimer. Yet another had begun to write and another to travel.

Others were doing volunteer or mission work. Virtually all were reading more, rocking more, walking more, eating better—and above all else, experiencing what they described as "better health," even though their bodies were, in most cases, in the declining stages of life.

Barb and I met scores of men and women who were open to change—and experiencing it—who were beginning to discover the healing power of following their own God-given hopes and dreams and not merely obeying the dictates of others. They were beginning to discover their future—their destiny, if you would—but ironically at a time when the years ahead of them were limited. Some were even considering new careers—something they'd always dreamed of doing but hadn't, because they'd chosen another path or (perhaps better to say) followed a path chosen for them or expected of them.

In other words, many had spent a great portion of their life seeking to please others instead of seeking the path their Creator had charted for them. Oh, most of them made lots of money, wore the best clothes, drove big cars, had summer homes. But ultimately they lacked an inner peace.

I'm convinced that these people would tell you to begin *now* to discover and develop, to nurture and nourish, the path in life you were designed to walk—a path that will result in great satisfaction and health.

LIVING BY DESIGN

I believe with all my heart that each of us personally was created meticulously by a Master Designer. We exist for a reason, and we are loved by our Creator beyond our wildest imaginings. We are designed for a purpose. Jesus noted that he came to earth so that each of us "may have life, and have it to the full."

In talking about the beautiful benefits of a personal relationship with God, authors Frank Minirth, Paul Meier, Richard Meier, and Don Hawkins observe that "the believer has an opportunity to find meaning and purpose in his or her life." They write, "For believers, purpose and meaning in life is recognizing that we are not our own, but instead we belong to [(God]." They ask each of us this question: "Have you dedicated your life to him for whatever he wills?" If you have, "You will then discover your calling and internal identity as God's servant and ambassador and look for ever-increasing occupational opportunities that will allow you the most freedom in expressing who you are for the glory of God."

In a letter to the Christians in Rome, the apostle Paul wrote, "Therefore, I urge you, brothers, in view of God's mercy, to offer your bodies as living sacrifices, holy and pleasing to God—this is your spiritual act of worship. Do not conform any longer to the pattern of this world, but be transformed by the renewing of your mind." The Greek word *syschemmatizom,* translated as *conform,* means "to be molded by external forces," while *transformed* (*metamorphoom*—the root for our word *metamorphosis)* means "to be changed from the inside out."

When Jesus taught about food and clothing—the necessities of life—he said, "But seek first [God's] kingdom and his righteousness, and all these things will be given to you as well." If we want our lives to be infused with satisfaction, meaning, purpose, hope, and joy, the Bible tells us that it can only happen by knowing God personally and choosing to serve and please him daily—which is his purpose for us. In contrast, choosing to live outside of the purpose for which we were created inevitably results in a lack of wholeness, a shortage of passion, a deficiency of blessedness, and dissatisfaction—put simply, it results in "dis-ease."

The treatment of this type of dis-ease has two components. The first element we've already talked about, namely, coming to know God and developing a vital personal relationship with him. The second involves living out our God-given hopes and dreams in the context of our Creator's purpose for our lives.

In his book *The Power of Purpose*, Richard Leider points out, "Purpose is not a thing. It is never a static condition we can preserve. Purpose is a continuous activity, questions we ask over and over again. It's a process we live every day. It's a process for listening and shaping our life stories." Not only is finding your life story a key to achieving a high degree of health, discovering your role in God's story is critical as well. (For learning more about this, I recommend a marvelous resource by Kurt Bruner titled *The Divine Drama: Discovering Your Part in God's Story*.)

Derrick was a man who for most of his life had vision but no purpose. Thus he couldn't focus on the most important things that he needed to be doing. For the last two years of his life, he finally had both purpose and vision—he discovered his God-given hopes and dreams and began to live them out. If only he had started earlier.

A patient of mine in Bryson City, Derrick had been a successful and driven businessman, admired and respected by almost everyone in town. He seemed to have it all—power, prestige, and position. He was handsome and highly intelligent. He had the three "Bs" the world admires—beauty, brains, and bucks.

I had known about Derrick, even heard him give a talk at the Rotary club. He seemed to have it all together. One day he came to see me for a physical exam. I took an extensive history, examined him from head to toe, and then reviewed his lab results, X rays, and EKG results. I gave him what I thought was good news. He seemed to be in perfect shape—except for carrying a few too many pounds.

Derrick's response was surprising. "I hate my life. I hate my job. I hate my marriage. God forgive me, but I even hate my kids. I don't know what to do about it." As he told me this, his eyes filled with tears.

I sat down, and we talked a bit. Derrick was an agnostic, but he had come to a point in life when he felt a deep need to know if there was a God and if there was more to life than just getting and spending. I referred him to a local psychologist, who was also a pastoral counselor. They had several sessions together, but Dr. Larson told me later, "Derrick has decided not to change. He's chosen to stay on his current path."

Not long after this, Derrick moved to another city to take a more prestigious position with a larger company. We lost touch for about twenty years. Then, just two years ago, I was walking through an airport when I saw Derrick's wife approaching. We took some time to sit in a small café and catch up on what was going on in our lives.

"How's Derrick?" I asked. "And the kids?"

Joni was silent for a moment, then smiled sadly. "He passed away last year—at fifty-four years of age."

"What happened?"

"Walt, I think he worked himself to death. After we left Bryson City, he just climbed the corporate ladder. He was never at home. Our relationship fell apart. The kids grew to hate him, and they rebelled against me. Although he was miserable in his work, he just chose to continue in it—destroying himself and his family."

"I'm so sorry to hear that."

"Well, there was kind of a good ending," she confided.

"Kind of?"

"Yes." She paused for a moment and sipped her coffee. "About two years before he died, he realized that he—and we—were in terrible shape. A coworker began to share with him how he could have a personal relationship with God. Derrick decided to open himself up to that. The change was remarkable—almost instantaneous. He became involved in a small church and a men's Bible study group. The girls and I couldn't believe our eyes. In fact, for a while we thought he was acting. But as time went on, we knew it was real. He asked us to forgive him—which I must admit was kind of difficult, especially for our oldest daughter. But eventually we did, and he moved back home. Then he shocked us."

"What happened?" I asked.

"He quit his job. He said he had always wanted to be a coach. He wanted to help kids. So he left his career behind and took a coaching position at the local YMCA."

"You could afford that?" I asked.

"Not really, but we decided to make it work. We had to sell our home and the expensive cars. We downsized in every way. But, Walt, we've never done a better thing. Derrick was a new man. He had found his purpose. He loved what he was doing, and he fell in love with me and the girls—perhaps for the first time."

"That must have been something to see!"

"It was. Then came the heart attack. We got him to the hospital, but he died the next day." Joni lowered her head and tears began to stream down her cheeks.

I handed her my handkerchief. She wiped her eyes and took a deep breath, then looked back at me. "The night before he died, we had some precious time together. He told me how much he loved me and the girls. He told me how sorry he was for all the harm he'd done. But, Walt, he was most sorry for some of the choices he had made earlier in life—choices that kept him from finding out sooner who he really was, what his true purpose was, what he was meant to do."

We talked for a few more moments, then left to catch our flights. As my plane lifted off the ground, I found myself remembering how Derrick had grappled with feelings of purposelessness and even despair. It had been heartbreaking for me not to get through to him when I was his doctor. I so wished I could have waved a magic wand and opened his eyes to his God-given potential and the joy a person has when living up to it. To not be able to do so was frustrating for me twenty years before—yet I was so pleased to learn that he'd at least known a couple of years of joy and purpose.

Sometimes even more frustrating is to watch my patients who have a personal relationship with God and who accept the biblical teachings, yet who still wonder, *What is my purpose? Why am I here? Where is true joy and satisfaction?* Most of these men and women believe that God created them and loves them, yet they still sense that they haven't uncovered God's plan for their lives—that they're not at the center of God's will. Most of these folks seem to feel that there's more to life than what they're experiencing. They wish they could be doing something else. Most don't feel significant or fulfilled. They are not at ease—they aren't whole and aren't experiencing blessedness. They are, in a word, diseased.

What did I prescribe for my patients who were in this quandary? What would I recommend for you? Three simple words: *Discover your destiny.* Begin the process of determining God's very personal plan for your life and take action to live it with gusto. How? I'd prescribe reading and studying the book *Discover Your Destiny* by Bill and Kathy Peel.

I've noticed, though, that most people have an inborn wariness of their own hopes and dreams. It's as though they believe that their Creator could not possibly want them to see their dreams come true. Like some of the folks I talked about in the last chapter, they simply do not see themselves as God sees them. And as a result, by not pursuing their hopes and dreams they forfeit many of the blessings and the deep fulfillment he longs to give them.

Take a Long Look in the Mirror

Before you read any further, take time to consider the following:

- Do I believe that I'm in the center of God's plan for my life?
- Do I experience joy and satisfaction in my life and work?
- Do I have a sense of partnering with God to bring him glory and to serve others?

Take time to write out in your journal your answers to these questions and any others that may come to mind. Don't be concerned if it takes you a while! It may raise some very uncomfortable issues. You don't need all the answers—just write down what God brings to mind. Then begin to think, meditate, and pray about what it is you really think God is calling you to do and and to be.

Finding your destiny—living out your hopes and dreams—is becoming what your Creator created you to become. God doesn't want you to be miserable! Rather, he wants you to experience joy and peace as you do the very things he created you to accomplish. Many people think that seeking God's will and inflating their spiritual wheel require them to *give up their dreams and pleasures.* In fact, nothing could be more unhealthy—or unbiblical!

Please hear me out. Men and women who choose to live their lives strictly in accordance with their own selfish desires are *not* becoming highly healthy people. Those who seek to gain God's assistance in fulfilling their own agendas simply will *not* find their true destiny or enjoy high degrees of health. Even those who choose to do what they were created to do, but do it for selfish reasons—for their own benefit and glory—also cannot become highly healthy people experiencing lasting satisfaction. It is only those who do what they were created to do—in a right relationship with their Creator and with the right motives (to glorify and please God while serving him and others)—who have the opportunity to become highly healthy.

Researchers are confirming what I'm prescribing, namely, that having a sense of purpose and meaning results in higher degrees of health. According to noted wellness promoter Don Ardell, "The research suggests that the wellest of the well possess the following qualities, to an uncommon degree: high self-esteem and a positive outlook; a foundation philosophy and a sense of purpose; a strong sense of personal responsibility; a good sense of humor and plenty of fun in life; a concern for others and a respect for the environment; a conscious commitment to personal excellence; a sense of balance and an integrated lifestyle." Another researcher points out that arthritis patients who have a sense of purpose and who believe in themselves and in the meaning of their lives are happier and more satisfied and serene.

In one study, half to two-thirds of children from incredibly difficult backgrounds overcame the odds and showed real resilience in transforming their lives. One way this resilience is measured is "having a sense of purpose and a belief in a bright future, including goal direction, educational aspirations, achievement motivation, persistence, hopefulness, optimism, and spiritual connectedness."

So how can *you* discover your destiny—your Creator's purpose for you? How do you get in touch with your God-given hopes and dreams—perhaps abandoned somewhere along life's path—and nurture them back to life? The first step is to recognize, name, and then follow your personal and God-created passion.

An article in a journal for dentists points out that commitment and passion are often different aspects of the same thing:

> Passion is doing something not just because you like doing it but because it will make a difference in the world in the longer term.... Just doing what you like because it provides a personal satisfaction will eventually become dull. There are only so many ways in which you can get satisfaction doing something for yourself. With passion, there is no limit to the number of ways in which satisfaction will come to you.

Here's another way to put it: Your God-created passion is not simply something you do; it's something you can't *not* do.

FOLLOW YOUR PASSION

Tim dropped out of high school—well, actually, he was kicked out. A person of great passion, he often expressed his emotions and his beliefs with his fists. After dropping out of school, he had a tough time keeping a job. In one year he was fired from over fifty jobs! (It's true—he counted them.) Finally he found one he could keep. He became a garbage man.

When I met Tim, he was *not* highly healthy. He was overweight, diabetic, and hypertensive, and he didn't sleep well. Perhaps worse, he was stuck in a job he hated. It paid the bills and kept food on the table—but he felt as though his life was wasting away, just like the garbage he pitched into the dump each day.

When I became Tim's physician (the city gave him his first medical insurance policy), I discovered an unusually witty and intellectually gifted man. He loved to read and could quote Dante and Shakespeare. Better yet, he was willing to work on becoming a highly healthy person. We began working on improving his nutrition and increasing his exercise. Some supplements and medications helped decrease the severity of his physical ailments. Tim began to work on his emotional, relational, and spiritual wheels by getting involved in a local faith community that accepted him with open arms. They loved him and taught him. They gave him a sense of personal value in the context of genuine community. He began a personal relationship with his Creator. In this group of fellow spiritual travelers, he also found his life partner, and they were married.

Over time, Tim was visibly becoming more highly healthy. Yet his soul was still restless. He knew that he was created for something, but he wasn't sure just what it was. My next job was to help direct him to the port of his passion. I told Tim that finding and fulfilling his passion was like a lost sea captain locating the North Star after a storm. Successful navigation simply meant finding his passion and steering his life by it. I told him that his passion would be his internal compass—placed there by his Creator. Identifying what made him feel passionate would help him discover God's will for his life.

By passion, I'm referring to a God-given, deep-seated longing for something—a divinely directed capacity to feel so deeply attracted to doing something that it becomes a source of power and momentum, something you cannot *not* do. This type of passion is a persistent and powerful guide toward our God-ordained destiny. It can be suppressed, but it takes energy—and doing so causes harm. Because a life-directing passion is placed in each person by God, *not* moving toward fulfilling this inner desire can only result in dissatisfaction, discontent, disappointment, and displeasure.

In *Alice's Adventures in Wonderland,* Lewis Carroll describes so clearly a life without passion or direction. Alice is talking to the Cheshire Cat. She says, "Would you tell me, please, which way I ought to go from here?" The cat replies, "That depends on where you want to go." Alice then reveals her lack of passion or direction by replying, "I don't much care." The wise old cat informs her, "Then it doesn't matter which way you go." Alice tries to add, "So long as I get somewhere." And the cat responds, "Oh, you're sure to do that."

Tim was definitely moving in a direction, but it was not the direction of his passion. My prescription was for him to get up early each morning for a week and take a walk alone, and as he did to begin asking his Creator to reveal his passion, his destiny, God's plan. I also encouraged him to gather input from his parents, siblings, friends, colleagues, boss, and pastor. I told him that this input should only be a starting point, but when combined with his own inner voice of intuition, he might begin to get some direction.

Tim agreed. After only his second walk, he called me at the office. "I've got it. I've got it!"

"What?" I asked.

"I want to teach. In fact, I want to teach on a college campus."

There were a lot of obstacles. Very likely his family wouldn't be support-ive—no one in his family had ever gone to college. He didn't have a high school diploma. He didn't have the money to go to college. But he had something much more important—his passion—and it began driving him to his destiny.

Over the next six years, Tim went to night school to get his GED and his two-year associate's degree, and then he graduated from college with a bache-lor of science degree in education. After college he was awarded a scholarship and a graduate teaching position. He completed his master's degree and then his Ph.D.! He came to my office with his diploma, and we danced—we actu-ally danced—together.

Today Tim is teaching at a university in the Midwest. He hasn't lost as much weight as I'd like him to, but he's healthier than most men and women I know. In fact, he's highly healthy. He's discovered his destiny. He exempli-fies what Joe Paterno, football coach at Penn State, once said: "Believe deep down in your heart that you're destined to do great things."

I agree with Thomas Edison: "If we all did the things we are capable of doing, we would literally astound ourselves." I'd alter his words a bit to say, "If we all did what we were destined to do, we would live astounding lives!"

Determine to Discover Your Destiny

Take time to jot down your passions in your journal. Make your list as long as necessary.

What do you long to do? What are your deepest desires? Write down the things you perceive are keeping you from following your passion. List every obstacle you can possibly imagine. What would it take to follow your passion? What support do you have? What would you need now and along the way?

Remember, our Creator specializes in the impossible. Miracles still happen—even today!

FACE YOUR PERSONAL OBSTACLES

Tim chose not to live in the status quo. He chose to discover and then follow his passion. He didn't give in to his or his family's unfounded fears. He didn't accept a discontented existence. He knew that wasn't what his Creator wanted for him. So he faced and overcame the obstacles—both internal and external—that threatened to hold him back. He lived out the insight of Helen Keller: "Life is either a daring adventure or nothing."

Recently Barb and I were visiting friends whose neighbor had a young golden retriever confined to the yard by an electronic fence. The fence had a buried cable that would cause a probe in the dog's collar to lightly shock the dog if she got too close to the underground wire. So she stayed in the yard. Safe, never straying, but always looking longingly at the edge of the bay that lapped up next to the property.

We were sitting on the back porch when some people came down the beach with their puppies. Exuberant in their energy, the puppies were chasing sticks being thrown into the water. The golden retriever's ears cocked forward and her tail wagged ferociously as she slowly crept up to the buried wire. She knew where she was called to be, and it was *not* within the safety of the yard. Her heart longed to join the puppies in the water she loved—the waves where she was meant to frolic.

We wondered if she would risk the momentary shock. Was the memory of the pain she had experienced in the past too scary? As the family slowly moved down the beach, the dog stayed in the yard. When the playful puppies were out of view, the retriever sunk down and literally moaned.

The next morning while out for a walk I met the dog's owner and shared our observations from the evening before. He laughed. "You know," he said, "we've had that wire turned off for several weeks now." I felt a pang of sadness. It was the pain of her past that was keeping that dog imprisoned—not free to be who she was created to be.

Perhaps you are like that dog. Afraid to venture out of your yard, afraid of being hurt yet again or of failing one more time. Yet miserable on the inside. Deep down you want to move out and move on. I want to offer you a prescription of hope: No matter what your age, it is never too late to become the person you were designed to be. In fact, if you want to be highly healthy, you *must* reach forward and upward to fulfill your God-given potential.

Why do so many people allow their dreams to be derailed? Why do so many settle for what comes along, too afraid to take a risk and step out onto new ground, even though they're miserable? Why do they deny their hopes and forego living out their destiny? I've heard many reasons—things I've come to realize are their own personal obstacles:

- "I feared failure."
- "I was afraid of rejection." (One man told me, with quivering chin and misty eyes, "I'm finally realizing that if I only do things that guarantee

I'll be 100 percent safe from rejection, then I'm probably not fulfilling a purpose that is greater than my own fears.")

- "I thought only a few special people have a true destiny—have true purpose." ("I made a mistake," one elderly patient told me. "Now I realize we all have a true destiny. I wish I'd learned this earlier.")
- "I feared disapproval and censure. I was scared to death of criticism." (A man in his late eighties, tears spilling from his eyes, told me, "My mother's criticism kept me from my dreams. Only recently did I step out from under her critique—and she died over forty years ago.")
- "I was too busy chasing the dreams of my parents rather than my own destiny."
- "I was just too tired. I was so busy selfishly building my career—doing my thing—that I not only missed my kids growing up, but I also missed God's best for me and for my family."
- "I stayed too isolated. I didn't get outside myself." (One man said, "By choosing to serve only myself and not my community, I was missing out on God's plan for my life. It was only when I began serving others that I really discovered who I was and what I was supposed to be doing.")

What Is Poisoning Your Passion?

In your journal, add other reasons that may be keeping you from following your passion. Take a few moments to consider your options. What would it take for you to move from where you are today to where you want to be? List at least two specific things you can do to get started. Then write down how and when you will start.

Ken was one young man who did live out his God-given hopes and dreams. Ken was a medical student who did a monthlong family medicine rotation in our practice. He lived with Barb and me in Bryson City, and he studied alongside me.

During one of our evening talks, I shared how Barb and I had dreamed of traveling in Europe. Rather than waiting for retirement, I worked hard to graduate from medical school early so I could use the available six months to travel and study in Europe. During that time we visited thirteen countries, and as students, we did so at a significantly lower cost than we could have later in life. We made several lifelong friends and learned lessons that proved priceless later on. For example, my first book, *Alternative Medicine* (coauthored with Dónal O'Mathúna) was based on the foundational education I received in natural medicines while traveling and studying in England and Germany.

As Ken listened to our experiences, his eyes lit up. He and his wife had also dreamed of going to Europe. But where, he wondered, would he get the time? The money? We discussed several strategies, and I encouraged him to talk to others and to begin to pray about this dream.

Ken finished medical school and completed his family medicine residency. He and his wife were feeling the call to become medical missionaries, but they weren't sure where to go. There were so many countries that needed the services they could provide. And they still had a dream to travel. After talking to others and seeking God in prayer, they began to dream not just about a trip to Europe but a trip around the world.

As they continued to dream and plan and pray, the details began coming together. They recently completed a trip around the world, visiting missionaries in many countries and cultures. Based on their travels, they now have a much greater sense of how God is calling them to spend their lives as medical missionaries. Ken is one man who will not look back at the age of eighty and say, "I wish I had followed my dreams and discovered my destiny."

Pick Your Passion

Pick one thing from your list—one passion—that you could accomplish if you would *just do it*. Decide *how* you will do this, and write it down in your journal. Decide *when* you will do this, and write it down in your journal. *Share your dream* and plan with someone you love—and begin to pray about your destiny.

KEEP HOPE ALIVE

Hope is a powerful antidote for anyone who needs an attitude adjustment—and so much of discovering our destiny has to do with attitude. Will we let our own negativity and fear keep us trapped? Or will we light the flame of hope and pursue our God-given desires—our vision—for our good and for his glory?

One medical review of the studies focused on hope concluded, "Investigators agree that hope is an important coping skill for patients. Hope is stronger than optimism and influences one's physical well-being." In other words, hope is essential to high degrees of health. Hope has been shown to have significant therapeutic value, whereas *demoralization* (defined as hope-lessness and meaninglessness) can significantly interfere with becoming highly healthy.

A study of diabetics demonstrated a relationship between the meaning patients attributed to their illness and the seriousness of that illness. The positive attitudes of hope, motivation, and control (a sense of personal empowerment) all affected the behavioral and mental adjustments of persons living with diabetes. The study concluded that the more positive the patient's attitude toward the illness—the more hope a patient had—the better his or her mental and physical health outcomes. In short, hope makes a difference!

I learned from Eva that it's never too late to light the flame of hope. Eva had become addicted to tobacco products when she was a very young woman. She smoked because everyone she knew—her parents, her relatives, and *all* of her friends and colleagues—smoked. By the time I met her, she had severe emphysema. She also had a number of other chronic medical conditions, but the emphysema was her worst problem. Sadly, the disease was in its final stages. There was little I could do medically other than to keep her comfortable.

She was declining quickly, and we began planning for the end of her life—discussions that are never easy at first. But as the reality of death approaches, most patients come to accept it and sometimes even welcome it. Eva began her preparations.

Predicting death is extremely difficult for physicians. Sometimes we think it's a week or a month away, yet it doesn't come for a year; sometimes we think it's years away, yet it happens in days. But for Eva it did appear as though the end was defined in months. She had virtually no strength. She couldn't walk or carry out her daily living activities without the help of one or two others. She slept for long periods of time. She entered the hospital for what I was sure was her last stay there.

Then it happened. One of her daughters became pregnant—with the granddaughter Eva had always wanted. Eva made a rally that amazed the nurses, the consulting pulmonologist, and me. Her strength increased, but, even more important, her will to live was renewed. Within days she was released from the hospital, and she walked from the wheelchair to her husband's car with no assistance.

When I delivered the baby girl thirty-two weeks later, her grandmother was there to witness the miracle. She was radiant and beaming as she held her first grandchild in her arms. Her tears flowed freely when she learned that baby Eva would be named after her!

Six weeks later, little Eva's mother brought her to the office for a well-baby visit. That same afternoon the three of us attended Grandma Eva's funeral.

You might think this story unusual, but for most physicians it's commonplace. We've witnessed time and time again the impact of hope, dreams, and a strong sense of destiny on a patient's health—and on the living of life itself.

A vignette from the life of my friend Bob Garner provides another stellar example of the power of hope. Bob's initiation into the entertainment world was with the *Carol Burnett* and *Red Skelton* shows. From there he worked his way up the ladder to become an executive producer for Walt Disney Imagineering and Theme Park Films and then for Focus on the Family Films. His award-winning work has long been admired by many.

Bob grew up in the Asheville, North Carolina, area. He moved to California to pursue his dreams and destiny. His mother and father stayed back in the mountains in which they had raised their three boys. After Bob's mom died, Bob's dad seemed to lose his desire to live. His heart condition worsened, despite the very best medical care, and his health deteriorated rapidly.

Bob went to visit him as often as possible, and each time their relationship grew stronger. Bob never knew which visit might be his last with his dad. Finally the call came. His dad had suffered a severe heart attack and was in a coma. The doctors didn't expect him to live long.

Bob debated whether to go to his father's side immediately—or just wait and attend the funeral. He had already said good-bye to his dad. But Bob felt led to go back to Asheville as soon as possible. When he arrived at the hospice, his dad was still alive—though in and out of a coma and expected to die at any moment.

Bob entered his dad's room and sat at the bedside. He reached over to grasp his dad's cool hand. "Pop," he whispered, "I'm here."

Then to Bob's (and the nurse's) astonishment, his father, who hadn't talked for several days, opened his eyes, turned to face his son, and whispered back, "Bob, I've been waiting for you."

Indeed he had been. Bob's dad died peacefully the next day. Bob said, "My older brothers had been by Dad's side. It was as though Dad wouldn't let go until he had seen me—his youngest son—to make things complete."

Bob's last conversation with his dad is one of his most special memories—one of the most wonderful gifts his dad could have given him.

Having Trouble Finding Your True Purpose?

Try this simple exercise. For several days in a row, as you think about each day, ask yourself the following questions (writing the answers in your journal):

- What did I most dislike about today, and why?
- What would be the complete opposite of the things I disliked?
- What would I have liked to have done today?
- What was I called to do today?

Once you've written down your answers, think about the following questions: "What do people most value about me?" "What is most important to me in my work and in my personal life?" Listen for an honest response from your heart. Then record your impressions in your journal.

Take your time. Revisit these questions every day for a few weeks. If you can't answer a question, leave it for another day.

Having trouble finding your passion, your direction in life? Consider taking a walk and spending time alone—just you and your Creator. Ponder some of the principles we've discussed. Then, in a day or so, read this chapter again, slowly. Here's why: If you don't get this idea, you won't get the rest. And it will be very difficult for you to become a highly healthy person.

If this chapter makes some sense to you, don't expect it to make perfect sense—at least not right away. Let this information seep into your thinking. Meditate on it and pray about it. Why? Because a passionate sense of purpose and personal destiny is the foundation to higher levels of health. "Passion," says psychiatrist Boyd J. Slomoff, "is what can change choice into commitment. It is a guarantee of reward that is as everlasting as your participation."

We've now completed 80 percent of our reflections on the ten essentials of highly healthy people. I know the journey hasn't been easy. But the truth is this: no reward worth seeking and having is an easy one to obtain.

Most of what I've covered has involved your working with and on *yourself*. Now I'm going to shift gears a bit. Although there is much you can do to improve your personal health, it should be obvious that you also need medical expertise—a winning health care team. In the two concluding chapters, I'll deal with how you can customize your health care plan by becoming your own quarterback and teaming up with the best practitioners you can find.

CHAPTER ELEVEN

Be Your Own Health Care Quarterback

The Essential of Personal Responsibility and Empowerment

You have the right—and the obligation to yourself—to participate in the decisions that affect your health care." That's the advice of Dr. Isadore Rosenfeld, a distinguished professor of clinical medicine at New York Hospital, Cornell Medical Center, in New York City.

In a *Parade Magazine* article, Dr. Rosenfeld described what is happening in health care in the United States. "The truth is, medical care is rationed in this country," he wrote. "Physicians are spending less time with their patients. Many now work for insurance companies or managed care providers who have the last word on what tests or treatments they'll pay for. You may not even be told that there are better options than what you've been offered. So now, more than ever, you're essentially on your own when it comes to protecting your health and well-being."

Many of my patients, as well as those who have called in to my radio and television programs, tell me they feel baffled, even powerless, in the face of the myriad of health care options available, especially in the context of our managed care system today. They also seem confused over medical reporting in the media. As one caller told me, "One day they say a high-protein diet is healthy—

and the next day they say it's deadly. Who should I believe? Can't you doctors ever get the story straight?"

The issue, I told the caller, is not just the doctors. At least to some degree the issue also involves the caller herself. I told her that as long as she depended completely on others—even educated professionals—who might have a plethora of opinions about everything from aloe to zinc, from acupressure to Zen, from pap smears to cancer treatments, she was likely to become *more*, not less, confused.

Furthermore, the likelihood of increasing confusion is escalating dramatically. A tidal wave of medical information hits us every day—from our morning paper, to the national magazines, to the evening news and TV magazine shows, to the radio reports—not to mention the massive amounts of information available on the Internet. Many times we consumers have reports on medical studies days, even weeks, before the medical journals get to our doctors' offices.

My caller needed to begin to take control of her own health and do her own work toward becoming highly healthy. "I don't know if you're a football fan," I told her, "but let me give you an analogy I've shared with my patients for years: You need to become your own health care quarterback. You'll need a good primary care physician as your coach—someone who's a medical expert and willing to listen to you, to coach and advise you—sometimes even to fuss at you and push you.

"You may also need some specialists—assistant coaches. These coaches are trained in a specific aspect of the game. They know almost everything there is to know about the part of the body they're in charge of, but they can't see the entire game in the same way you and your coach can."

I paused, allowing time for the idea to take hold. The caller was quiet. "The best teams—the ones that win the most—have great quarterbacks working with great coaches. In your 'health game,' you need to learn how to call the plays. Does that make sense?"

The caller's response, sadly, was not atypical. She sighed deeply and retorted, "Well, sonny, that's *your* job, not mine!" She hung up.

This caller wanted a doctor to tell her what to do and to prescribe the best treatment for her. But the changes that are occurring in health care mean that you, the patient, must take charge of your health care—become your own *health care quarterback.*

I suspect that many readers may find the idea of taking responsibility for their own health care surprising—or even wrong. A friend told me, "I like the idea of *participating* in making the best health care decisions for myself. I agree that I need to do my homework and focus more on prevention. But I'm not a medical expert, nor do I want to be. You doctors go to medical school for years to gain the expertise I desperately need when I have a health problem."

If these are your thoughts, then rest assured, I understand. But there is a distinct difference between expecting (or even demanding) a physician to make a decision for you—without your educated input—and choosing a caring physician who will work in partnership with you to educate you, empower you, and enable you, while expecting you to participate as much as you can in your health care responsibilities and decision making.

Be sure you understand, though, that it doesn't take nearly as much skill or time for a physician to tell you what to do as it does for him or her to educate and guide you, to help you decide both what you *should* do and what you *want* to do. This is professional expertise at its best.

A friend who read this chapter wrote me the following note:

> *Sure, point me to some interesting Internet sites where I can gain a better understanding of my condition, listen to my theories based on my totally informal (and perhaps irrelevant and misleading) research as a layperson, help me understand my options—but do so as the educated and experienced medical professional I'm paying you to be. I do want to hear my doctor's advice and opinions and especially recommendations regarding my particular condition. I'm not qualified to sort through all the options myself and make a sound medical decision. I need an expert to inform me about the whole process and recommend the best treatment options. This is the doctor's job, as far as I'm concerned.*

To my friend I say, "I totally agree!" That's exactly what your doctor should do—make recommendations that explain in clear terms the nature of your medical problem and what treatment options you have. The doctor should also advise you on what is normally the best plan for your particular medical problem. Note, though, the words *recommendations* and *options*. Your doctor needs to give you all the information you need, then let *you* make the final decision on what play to call.

As you learn how to become your own health care quarterback, I encourage you to do at least two things: (1) Be more proactive and take more responsibility than you probably took in the past, and (2) find a personal physician who will be your health care coach.

You *don't* want a coach who will overwhelm you with data, research conclusions, and divergent opinions—and then leave you to make your own "health care bed." If you took the required time to learn all that is knowable about any one serious medical condition, you could easily be even more diseased by the time you sorted through the endless medical opinions. Not to mention that you're not trained or experienced enough to do so! But as Dr. Rosenfeld points out, "Knowledge is power. You should have as much information as possible about your condition—and your rights—so that you have the confidence to share in the decisions that affect *your* health, the quality of *your* life, and survival itself. The better prepared you are to ask informed questions, the better your chances of receiving optimum medical care."

Look for a physician who will guide you in exploring the best possible options regarding your health care and treatment, then *recommend* to you what would, in the doctor's professional opinion, be your best options but who will then ultimately let *you* make the choice.

Listen to me carefully. I am *not* saying that you must become a medical expert in order to have any hope of becoming highly healthy. Of course not. What I am saying is this: When you actively participate in your care—in partnership with a physician who encourages such teamwork—you are operating according to the best model of medicine, the one most likely to result in your becoming highly healthy.

Another caveat: In the case of emergencies, the model I'm proposing clearly isn't tenable. If you have a serious laceration, if you've suffered a heart attack, if you've been injured in a car accident, you're in immediate need of a doctor who is both well trained and experienced. A prolonged discussion of options isn't necessary—or sometimes even possible. But for the majority of your medical care—for example, when you have a potentially lifelong chronic health problem or when you need to sort through preventive medicine options—then it's to your advantage to learn how to be your own health care quarterback under the guidance of a good health care coach.

Participating in your health care decisions is not an easy job. In fact, it's a pretty tall order. Here's at least part of what it entails:

- Learn of all of the possible treatment options for your condition—each with its own risks, benefits, and costs.
- Know how long the treatment(s) you and your doctor choose should take to work.
- Understand, as completely as possible, the goal of each of the treatments you and your doctor choose.
- Learn how to tell if the treatment is succeeding or failing.
- Learn your health care rights.
- Get answers to your many questions.
- Learn tips to make the health care system work in such a way that it will help you keep or regain the highest degree of health possible.

A tough job, yes—but doable. For over twenty years it was what I taught my patients to do. I'm delighted to report that the majority succeeded magnificently. In fact, because of their work, I was a better doctor. They'd bring me information about new treatment options I didn't know about. Their work allowed us to be strong health care *partners*. I'm convinced that these patients are more highly healthy as a result of our doctor-patient relationship because they were willing to learn the steps outlined above.

So what is job number one in becoming your own health care quarterback? Finding a terrific health care coach—your personal physician. Keep in mind that there is no way to accomplish the above tasks if your doctor (or his or her staff) is unwilling or unable to do so because of managed care or other restraints.

Too many patients let someone else make major decisions for them. Remember the caller I mentioned as I began this chapter? She made it clear that she had no interest in this kind of approach to health care. She wanted to hire someone to be both her health care coach and quarterback. She was demanding that someone care for her *completely*—by making all of her decisions for her. And, sadly, she'll have absolutely *no* problem finding this kind of doctor.

But she *will* have a problem: There's a high probability she won't be as healthy as she could be. You simply can't delegate *all* of your health care responsibilities and decisions to "the experts." Doctors of highly healthy patients know that there are *many* things they cannot do for their patients; they are fully aware that patients must take some responsibility for their own health care—especially when it comes to the issues discussed in this book. These physicians understand that patients have to play a central role in any strategy developed toward the goal of healthier living. And the best doctors want to equip and empower their patients to become their own health care quarterbacks.

I recently spoke with a caller to my radio program who told me he had been crippled with an inflammation of the foot—called plantar fasciitis—for over six months. The pain was keeping him from exercising, and as a result he gained considerable weight and began suffering from lower back pain. Keith complained that his HMO was slow to respond to his needs and desires.

It became clear rather quickly that at no time had Keith sought to take control of his own health. To all appearances he had never even considered that an option. Instead, he let the system take care of him—which it did poorly. Keith simply didn't know his rights as a patient.

Keith had violated several principles of being a highly healthy person—and was accelerating his aging and disease in the process. He saw his doctor as the boss—both coach and quarterback—and himself as the water boy who was supposed to do whatever he was told. He never made an effort to learn about any treatment options for his condition. He didn't even understand the goal of the one treatment he *had* tried, so he didn't know whether it was succeeding or failing.

Although my time with him was limited, I outlined several common treatment options for his condition—most of them simple and inexpensive.

Keith was surprised. "Why didn't the other doctor tell me these things?"

"Did you ask?" I inquired.

There was a pause, then, "Uh—no."

"That's an important first step," I said. "Ask the doctor about the diagnosis and the treatment options. If the doctor doesn't have the time to review the treatment options, then you can either make another appointment to discuss it or ask if a nurse can explain the options to you. For any treatment you choose, be sure to ask what to expect—how long the treatment should take before it starts working, what you should do if it's not working as expected, whether you should be rechecked and, if so, when. Is this making sense?"

"It is. In fact, I'm embarrassed to admit that it just sounds like common sense."

"It *is* common sense," I said. "But it's easy to forget to ask these things when you're in the middle of a hustling and bustling medical office."

"But what if my doctors don't want to give me this type of care?"

"Good question," I replied. "Fire them."

"Fire them?" Keith exclaimed. "Can I do that?"

"Yes. Even in an HMO plan you can usually do that."

WHY GO TO ALL THE TROUBLE? DOESN'T DOCTOR KNOW BEST?

The truth is—no, a doctor doesn't always know best. It's *your* responsibility to surround yourself with a group of health care players who not only have the knowledge to provide the care you need but also will take their signals from you.

You may be feeling a bit like my friend who informed me that most people she knows would have a hard time getting a doctor to stay in a room long enough to provide this kind of information and guidance. "Most office visits are over in fifteen minutes or less," she said, "and there's little the patient can do about it." To that I would simply say that to get the care you want and deserve, you must know that such care is available, then take steps to find it. You must ask for this type of care and expect to receive it.

My friend, along with many other people, had chosen to tolerate a physician who did not provide this type of care—even though a number of doctors in her town gave exactly the kind of care I encourage patients to seek. She chose *not* to seek the best care. To be your own health care quarterback, you're going to have to do some work, take some responsibility, and perhaps make some significant changes in your approach to your health care.

"But doesn't the doctor know what's best for me?" you ask. My answer is, "Not necessarily." No one—not even your physician—knows you as well as you know yourself. No one is better qualified and able to make a final medical decision for you than you are.

When I shared this perspective with one of my friends, he said, "Whoa, Walt, you'd better be careful. The words *able* and *qualified* may not be appropriate here. I may *know* a lot about my own body, and I'd surely want my doctor to take seriously my own perceptions. However, if I could figure out how to make the best decisions about my treatment—to say nothing of coming up with the diagnosis—then I wouldn't need a doctor, except perhaps to do a technical procedure like surgery. I may be *able* to make decisions about my health care, but I'm not *qualified* to make medical judgments and determinations. That's why I wish my doctors would do so—and I want to be able to trust them to make *good* judgments."

"Actually we're saying the same thing," I told him.

He looked bewildered.

"The doctor *should* be the one to diagnose your problem. The doctor *should* be the one to make medical judgments and determinations and then distill these into priorities and recommendations. Your doctor's job is to make sure you are informed and prepared. Here's the deal: For most nonemergency medical decisions, the doctor may not be the best one to make the decision. That's *your* job. The doctor's job is to guide you as you make your decision. *You* are the most qualified and able to make the final decision of what's best for you. Does that make sense?"

He nodded. "I think so." Then he paused a moment to rub his chin and think about what I had said. "You know, this is a really different way of looking at health care. I've never thought of it this way."

"But it *is* a highly healthy way to think."

He smiled.

Think about it for a moment. Would you agree that there is *no* single medical decision that is right for all persons of all genders at all ages and at all times? Of course you would. Every medical decision is unique—and should be unique. *You* are unique. Therefore, you should be involved in—and ultimately responsible for—the decisions made by and for you.

Are You Willing to Become Your Own Health Care Quarterback?

Contemplate what I've said in the last few pages. Does it make sense to you? If this is not the kind of medical care you're getting now, is it the kind of care you desire? If so, what steps do you need to take? Do you need to make an appointment with your doctor to talk about this kind of care and to see if he or she would encourage and enable such care? If your doctor is not willing to provide this kind of care, are you willing to make a change and actively seek this kind of care? If not, why not?

Consider the following example of the kind of doctor-patient relationship that generally results in higher levels of health for the patient. Sem, a devout Jehovah's Witness, was my patient for more than fifteen years. We had significant theological differences, and over these differences we agreed to disagree.

Born around 1920, Sem had grown up believing that "doctor knows best." Yet, as he matured in age and wisdom, he began to feel that it just wasn't true. He had heard of the increasing number of medical errors made by health care providers, especially in hospital settings. He had friends who had been prescribed the wrong medicine—or the wrong dose of medicine—and had been harmed. In fact, his wife, Mary, had been given a wrong medication in the hospital and had suffered a terrible effect. Sem had felt awful that he had allowed it to happen without asking any questions before or after. He knew he could have prevented the medication error if he had just asked a few questions—What are you giving her? Why is she getting this medication? What can we expect as it works in her body?

I met Sem in the middle of a medical predicament. He had seen his regular primary care physician for a routine annual checkup. During the standard digital rectal exam for a man of seventy (Sem's age), the physician noted that not only was Sem's prostate enlarged but there was a small, hard nodule in it. Wanting to rule out cancer, the doctor referred Sem to a surgeon. While Sem wondered about other options, he was afraid to ask. Hearing the word *cancer* had scared him to death. *And,* he thought, *doesn't the doctor know best?*

Sem's PSA test (the Prostate Specific Antigen blood test used to detect prostate cancer) was only slightly elevated; nevertheless, a subsequent biopsy by a urologist showed an early-stage prostate cancer.

The urologist told Sem there was only one choice to cure the cancer—surgery. "We need to do it quickly. I'll have my nurse schedule you for next week."

As scared as he was, Sem was more scared *not* to ask some questions. "What type of surgery?"

"We call it radical prostatectomy. I'll make an incision in your lower abdomen and take out the prostate gland. We should get all the cancer, and it should cure you."

The word *radical* struck Sem as—well—*radical.* Now he was even more concerned. He'd heard that surgery could do some damage "down there." That he might never . . . "Are there any complications with that kind of surgery?"

The doctor sighed and rolled his eyes. Sem said later that the urologist seemed to be in a hurry and that these questions obviously annoyed him. "Well, *any* surgery can result in abnormal bleeding, infection, or scarring. With any surgery you can have a reaction to medications or even the anesthesia— and there is an extremely remote chance of dying during or after the surgery. But if you want this cancer cured, then I need to operate."

Sem's commitment to his religion would not allow him to accept a blood transfusion, so the risk of bleeding was a concern to him—but not nearly as big a concern as the risk of dying on the operating table. Sem felt trapped. "Aren't there any other options?" he asked.

The surgeon told Sem that the radical surgery was the only way he could guarantee a cure.

"If I survive the surgery, are there any side effects afterward?"

Only then did the surgeon explain that many patients of other doctors had experienced impotence and urine leakage, but he assured Sem that *his* patients rarely had such problems.

Sem knew he didn't want to rush into a decision that day. "Can't we wait a bit so I can think about this and decide?"

"The longer you wait," the surgeon warned, "the more likely that this thing will grow and take your life." He said he had an opening for surgery in two days, then suggested Sem and his wife return the next day so all the arrangements could be made.

"Can I pray about it a bit?"

According to Sem, the surgeon looked even more irritated. He glanced at his watch, then at the ceiling. Then he said, "Sem, if we don't get this thing out, and get it out quick, you won't *have* a prayer."

When Sem asked about getting a second opinion, he said he thought the surgeon's eyes "were gonna pop right out of his head."

"Look here," the surgeon retorted, "the only reason you'll need a second opinion is if you don't trust me. And if you can't trust me, we can't have the type of doctor-patient relationship we need. So if you need another opinion, you go get it—but get it from your next doctor!"

The surgeon turned on his heel and left the room, slamming the door behind him.

After Sem got dressed, he walked alone to the waiting room. Mary stood to meet him and could plainly see his distress.

"Didn't go well, Sem?"

"Mary, he wants to put me under the knife day after tomorrow. And he doesn't want me to get another opinion. What do you think?"

"Sem," she answered, placing her hand reassuringly on his arm, "if you need a second opinion—or a third or a fourth—then you get it."

Sem and Mary left the office, never to return.

Both of Sem's health care providers had, in my opinion, failed Sem. Neither his primary care physician nor the urologist had told him of a number of reasonable options available to a sixty-year-old man with early-stage prostate cancer—treatments such as external beam radiation, internal radiation (brachytherapy, or "seeding"), cryotherapy (using liquid nitrogen to freeze and destroy the cancer), or "watchful waiting" (doing nothing).

Neither doctor told him about the risks, benefits, and costs of these options. Nor had they provided any handouts that clearly and simply explained these. They hadn't directed him to any number of excellent Internet sites that contain this information—along with pictures and illustrations—including the Websites of internationally recognized medical centers such as Harvard, Mayo, and Johns Hopkins.

Neither doctor had told Sem of the genuine risks of surgery (such as long-term erectile dysfunction, which occurs in as many as 60 percent of patients who undergo prostate cancer surgery, and urinary incontinence, which occurs in as many as 10 percent of surgery patients). The urologist was a surgeon who recommended what he knew best—surgery—and probably overstated the excellent results his patients experienced.

Studies show, not surprisingly, that when it comes to options for prostate cancer treatment, the recommendation you get generally depends on the specialist you see. The *Journal of the American Medical Association* reported on a survey of urologic surgeons (urologists) and radiation therapists (radiation oncologists), which revealed that a majority of each group would primarily recommend the treatment they provide. For example, 93 percent of the surgeons believed that prostatectomy (surgical removal of the prostate) offered the best cancer control, even though they admitted it was more likely to cause life-altering side effects. On the other hand, 72 percent of the radiation therapists believed that external beam radiation was just as effective as surgical removal.

So who is telling the truth to their patients—the urologists or the radiation oncologists? According to the study's author, Peter Albertsen, M.D., chief of urology at the University of Connecticut, they both are. He's convinced that both groups of doctors were being honest. Why? Because, he says, there's no compelling evidence that one type of treatment is better than the others.

This study, along with many others, simply underscores that if a doctor gives you only one recommendation, it's usually the one he or she is most comfortable with. However, it almost certainly is not the *only* option. And it's possible that it may not be the one that's best for you.

So what did Sem do? Someone recommended that he talk to me. When I saw him, I described all of the options—the risks, benefits, and costs of each. I told him where he could gain more information. But first I reassured Sem and Mary that they had time to make a wise decision and that no matter what choice they made, the chances of his dying from this cancer were very low. "In fact," I told them, "over 90 percent of the men who die over the age of ninety—and who die from something other than prostate cancer—had a prostate cancer growing in them that they didn't even know about. It tends to be a very slow-growing cancer—so we have time on our side."

As these facts sunk in, I could see the apprehension on Sem's face dissolve. "Let me have my nurse, Tish, give you some information on prostate cancer from the National Cancer Institute and the American Cancer Society," I said. "Feel free to give them a call at their toll-free phone number. They'd be happy to send you as much information as you need. And let's schedule a follow-up appointment to talk a bit more, OK?"

Both Sem and Mary nodded. Before they left, I made one last recommendation. "Sem, I'd encourage you to visit with and obtain the counsel of some of the older, wiser men in your faith congregation." He and his wife seemed shocked.

"You're giving me a funny look," I said. "What are you thinking?"

"Well, I've *never* had a doctor, particularly a Christian doctor, recommend that I talk to my elders at the Kingdom Hall," Sem answered.

I shared this timeless advice from the Bible: "Is any one of you sick? He should call the elders of the church to pray over him and anoint him with oil in the name of the Lord." And then as we stood at the end of our visit, I said, "Sem, I want you to know something about me. The most important relationship in my life is my personal relationship with God. He has not only changed me from the inside out, but he has also changed the way I practice medicine. He's taught me how essential it is that I talk to him about everything I do. I believe in the power of prayer. Sem, would it be okay if I pray for you right now?"

Both Sem and Mary looked surprised but nodded their assent. I prayed, "Dear God, I can't even begin to imagine how frightening this news about prostate cancer is—or how complex all these decisions must seem. But in the Bible you tell us that if we ask for wisdom, you will give it to us. So today I ask for wisdom for me and for Sem and Mary. Help us make the right decisions. Amen." After that day, no appointment with Sem came to an end without his asking for prayer. Our faith traditions were different, but our humanity in all of its frailty and need was a fertile common ground.

Before Sem and Mary left the office that day, my nurse, Tish, spent time with them to answer any questions. She asked if they wanted the names and phone numbers of several patients who had faced a similar diagnosis and had gone through the process of making these tough decisions. Each of these men (and their wives) had previously consented—enthusiastically, I might add—to help other men who faced this kind of difficult decision. Mary and Sem took the names of two couples to call.

It took two additional appointments to answer all of their questions. Each time they came back, they were armed with more information. Mary had called the National Cancer Institute and the American Cancer Society. The more they learned, the more concerned they became about the recommendation for surgery they had received previously.

At the end of their third appointment we came to a defining moment. "Dr. Larimore," Mary hesitated, looking at her feet, "I know that what I'm learning by reading and by calling these organizations agrees a whole lot with what you're saying, but the specialist we saw . . . " Her voice trailed off.

I understood her concern. Both their primary care doctor—whom they had known for years—and a well-respected specialist in treating prostate cancer had recommended one particular option; here I was, virtually unknown to them, recommending something else.

"If I were in your shoes," I explained, "I'd feel the same way. How in the world can you sort through these different recommendations and come to a wise decision?"

They both nodded.

"Here's an idea: You could get an opinion from the team at the cancer center. It means driving to the city, but they'll have several specialists who will see you. You'll be able to ask your questions and learn as much as you want. They wouldn't be doing the actual therapy—unless that's what you want—so you should get fairly objective information. After you see them, let's get together for another visit."

They made an appointment to get yet another opinion from a world-class cancer team in a nearby city. They saw a bevy of cancer experts, including a urologist who shared with them several surgical options; a radiation oncologist who was knowledgeable about several forms of external and internal radiation; and a medical oncologist who could counsel them about medical options—including watchful waiting. They also saw a psychologist and a chaplain who explained how cancer and these various therapies could affect them emotionally, relationally, and spiritually.

Sem called me to tell me that he was planning to visit with a doctor who had treated more prostate cancer patients with an experimental form of cryotherapy than any other doctor in the world. Although his insurance covered the consultation, it wouldn't cover this type of treatment. Sem and Mary were growing in their role as health care quarterbacks.

During the month or so that it took to obtain these consultations, Mary was hard at work teaching Sem to become Internet-savvy. I referred them to a number of Websites—sites I knew would provide reliable medical information—so that they could become lay experts in prostate cancer. Sem and Mary worked hard on all the assignments and became effective health care quarterbacks. And in the end they came to a decision. Sem chose watchful waiting.

At this writing, Sem is in his early eighties. He's more than ten years past his day of decision. His cancer is still there—still small—but it has *not* migrated to other parts of his body. His PSA level is unchanged. For the first few years after his diagnosis, he continued to see me (every three months) and a urologist (every six months). When it was clear that his cancer was very slow-growing, the urologist quit seeing him, and from then on I did a checkup every six months—along with a prayer!

Sem and I formed a great relationship. I began to work with him on some of his other physical concerns. He changed his diet, reducing his intake of saturated fats (which may contribute to prostate cancer) and increasing his intake of lycopene-containing vegetables, especially tomato sauce (which may help in the prevention and treatment of prostate cancer). He also takes a couple of vitamin and dietary supplements that some studies suggest may slow or reverse the growth of prostate cancer.

I don't know whether Sem's decision was right for most men in his situation—but it *was* the right decision for him. It was a decision he and his wife made with a great deal of confidence because of all the information they had gathered. Sem took control of his health care and, through the experience of the disease of cancer, became and remains highly healthy.

HOW TO TAKE CHARGE OF YOUR HEALTH CARE

What can you do to take charge of your health care? Especially if your doctor acts like the surgeon who tried to rush Sem to the operating room?

In today's health care system, many patients feel they're pretty much on their own when it comes to finding out about their illness. One of the reasons is that some doctors choose not to give their patients the information they need to be able to make wise and informed decisions.

For example, a recent study supported by the Agency for Healthcare Research and Quality discovered that doctors often do not do enough to help their patients make informed decisions. The study concluded that uninvolved and uninformed patients are less likely to accept the doctor's choice of treatment and less likely to do what they need to do to make the treatment work.

One health care writer who reviewed this chapter told me, "I think *most* physicians fail their patients, as you have described in Sem's case. So what's a patient to do?"

They need to do what Sem did. The key steps that Sem took mirror exactly the template I recommend to anyone who wants to work successfully with a health care provider to make medically reliable and biblically sound choices about their health. Following the G-U-E-S-T acrostic will increase your skills as a health care quarterback:

G = Get the facts.
U = Understand the different layers of health care.
E = Explore treatment options.
S = Seek wise spiritual counsel.
T = Take a personal inventory.

G = Get the Facts

Always begin your journey to health by asking your health care provider for a thorough summary of the issue at hand. Here are several questions to consider asking:

- What is my diagnosis?
- How certain are you that your diagnosis is correct?
- Could this be any other disease or condition besides the one being considered?
- What are the possible causes of my condition?
- What other symptoms might be expected or are usually seen?
- What tests or assessments are recommended for me? What will they cost? Will they be covered by my insurance?
- Where can I learn more about this disorder? Are there any Internet sites you would recommend? Any books you would recommend? Do you have any patient-education materials you could give me?
- Do you have other patients with the same condition who will share with me what they've learned and experienced?

Tips to Help You Get the Facts

If your appointment time with your health care provider is brief, reschedule a longer appointment to discuss your concerns. Bring a list of all the questions you have. Also consider bringing along your spouse or a trusted friend to listen, make notes, and ask questions. If your health care provider can't or won't spend the time with you that you desire, seek the opinion of one who will. This is your right and, in my opinion, your responsibility.

Double-check everything you hear and learn. If it's the truth, you'll be able to find documentation from several sources. If the sources conflict, then ask your personal physician to help you sort out the contradictions.

At this stage of dealing with your health care concerns, your emphasis should be on how to gather useful and reliable information. It's your job to become educated about your disease or disorder.

U = Understand the Different Layers of Health Care

There are several levels of the health care system from which you can gain care and information.

Primary Care

The first and most basic level of medical care is called *primary care.* Family physicians, pediatricians, and general (or primary care) internists commonly provide this care. These doctors are generalists who are trained to diagnose and treat more than 90 percent of the problems you may have.

However, there are still scores of conditions they may not have the training, experience, or time to treat. Most primary care physicians (PCPs) are eager to help you find the kind of specialty care you need. If they *can* provide the care, but you want a second or third opinion, most are happy—and *all* should be happy—to help you obtain those opinions.

For most patients, the best choice for a health care coach and advocate will be a primary care physician.

Secondary Care

These physicians are typically called *specialists.* They tend to care for a single organ system. For example, cardiologists care for problems of the heart and blood vessels, and neurologists care for problems of the brain, spinal cord, and nerves. Specialists are highly trained to care for problems in their limited area of expertise. For some patients, because of their type of health problem, the best choice for a health care coach or advocate is a specialist. Examples might include a woman's gynecologist, a heart patient's cardiologist, or a senior citizen's gerontologist.

Tertiary Care

For those problems that occur rarely or for treatments that are new, a person is best treated in the large medical centers usually associated with medical schools, research centers, or residency training programs. These centers care for the sickest of the sick. While a primary care physician might see one case of a particular disease in years of practice, a medical center's physicians may well have treated many each year. They also conduct research and are usually up-to-date with the newest treatments, as well as any experimental treatments.

For most people with health problems, it is reassuring and empowering to know there are experts with experience in treating their ailments. But I also understand that for some this system feels overwhelming and intimidating.

I recall a very frail elderly woman who simply did not feel up to the task of sorting through all the information. She had neither the interest nor the stamina. Since Georgia couldn't be her own health care quarterback, we needed to find one for her. I asked her about family, friends, neighbors, and folks at church. "Nope," she said. Her family had all moved away—and she didn't want to move to where they lived. She lived on a farm—no neighbors there. And she didn't go to church or synagogue. So there were no obvious candidates.

I explained to Georgia that she needed someone to help her, then asked if she wanted help to find someone.

She did.

By her next appointment, I had found, through a local church, a group of vivacious women Georgia's age who agreed to visit her twice a week—to bring lunch and to be her health care quarterbacks. Meals on Wheels agreed to deliver lunch five days a week. I talked to the man who would deliver her meals. He agreed to try to spend a little extra time with her each day.

I wish you could have seen the transformation in this patient! The "budding biddies," as they affectionately called themselves, took on their role with gusto. One or more of them brought Georgia to each of her doctor appointments. They fussed and fumed—and most of all cared.

I watched Georgia come alive before my eyes. In fact, through the years, *each* of these women, including Georgia, became more and more healthy. They were frail; they had many medical problems. But their health wheels inflated and became more balanced.

Georgia had felt intimidated and overwhelmed at what was to her a massive and scary health care system. Yet we found a way to overcome her fears (not to mention the restrictions of her insurance plan). Her surrogate quarterbacks scored the touchdowns, and Georgia won the game!

E = Explore Treatment Options

Whenever possible, obtain complete information on the risks, benefits, and costs of each suggested treatment option. Ask every health care expert you see, "What are *all* the potential treatments available to me, and how do you suggest we analyze them in order to come up with my best treatment option?"

Ask how your condition can be expected to progress with treatment—and without treatment. Even for the most commonly recommended options, ask the provider, "Will you discuss with me all the possible risks and benefits of what you are recommending? What will it cost? Of these costs, how much will I need to pay?"

Many providers aren't used to caring for people who are their own health care quarterbacks. Some may seem bothered by these kinds of discussions. If your doctor seems bothered or distracted, consider saying, "Doctor [or therapist or spiritual counselor], you seem distracted [busy, bothered]. Would there be a better time to schedule with you to discuss my concerns?"

When one of my friends asked a question like this of her doctor, she was told, "I'm not sure I have the time for this type of thing."

"No problem," she calmly replied. "Can you suggest another doctor who does?"

Her doctor smiled. He got the point. From then on, he made the time for her. But if he hadn't, she was prepared to go elsewhere to obtain the health care information she needed.

How to Change Doctors in an HMO

You may be thinking, *But my HMO won't allow me to change doctors more than once a year. I feel stuck!* Fortunately, that's not true.

Although most HMOs and some managed care plans only allow patients to *freely* change their doctor once (or sometimes twice) a year, that is not the case if you are dissatisfied with your doctor. Just call the insurance company or HMO. Explain your problem and why you need to change doctors. Most companies are not only understanding but also quite helpful to patients in accomplishing a change.

Resources on Navigating the Managed Care System

When I started my medical training over twenty-five years ago, most people in the United States had what was called *indemnity insurance coverage,* which allowed you to go to any doctor or hospital. The indemnity insurance would pay a large portion of the bill; the patient would pay a small portion.

Today, more than half of all Americans who have health insurance are enrolled in some kind of managed care plan—a plan organized both for providing medical services and for paying for them. A wide variety of such plans exist. Just a few of the more common types include preferred provider organizations (PPOs), health maintenance organizations (HMOs), and point-of-service (POS) plans.

While you may have heard these terms before, do you know what they mean? Do you know how they differ—and what the differences mean to you? Do you know how to navigate through these differences and all the various complexities?

To be a competent health care quarterback, you need help. One of the best resources is a document titled "Choosing and Using a Health Plan." This resource covers such questions as, What are my health plan choices? How do I compare health plans? How can I get the most from my plan? What if I have to go to the hospital? What about preexisting conditions? How do I choose a doctor?

You can download this valuable resource from the United States Agency for Healthcare Research and Quality via my Website at www.highlyhealthy.net.

What If My Doctor and I Don't See Eye to Eye?

Here are some things you can do when you don't understand or agree with your doctor's recommended course of treatment:

Don't be afraid to ask your doctor (or nurse) questions. Make sure you understand the recommendation and the reasons behind it. Usually there are excellent reasons for the treatment plan, but you have the right to know and understand the reason(s). Feel free to ask about any possible alternative treatments. If you forget to ask a question, call your doctor's nurse when you get home, or broach the subject with your doctor the next time you visit the office.

Seek a second opinion. It never hurts to get more than one opinion about the best course of treatment for your specific problem. It's your right to have the information you need to make a wise decision. If your doctor is uncomfortable with your desire to get a second opinion, then I think you should be uncomfortable with your doctor. You can always ask the folks at your health plan how to get a second opinion and whether the plan will pay for it. Usually it will.

Know that you have a right to change doctors if you consistently find yourself at odds with your physician. In most health plans, you may choose a new primary care physician at any time by contacting the health plan.

If you ever suspect your doctor has withheld proper medical care or treated you inappropriately, first discuss it with your doctor or one of the doctor's staff members. If you aren't satisfied, call your health plan. Most have a member services department. Ask to speak with a patient advocate whose job it is to help you resolve such problems. If necessary you can speak to your health plan's medical director or a board of doctors who do not belong to the plan. If you're still not satisfied, call your employer. Your employer may be able to help you resolve a problem or help you decide whether to file a grievance with the health plan. Finally, know that you can contact your state department of insurance or the state medical society to file a grievance.

S = Seek Wise Spiritual Counsel

Spiritual guidance and counsel, especially if you're facing a life-threatening situation, is a critical component of your health care team approach. If your congregation has elders, make an appointment to see them. Many elders are comfortable with and excited about this type of ministry. They may ask you some challenging questions about your spiritual health. They are often able to give you wise counsel and certainly will be able to pray with and for you. They may also be able to give you the names of others who have wrestled with the same problem(s). And if you need the help of a surrogate health care quarterback, they may be able to assist you.

If your faith community does not have elders, schedule a visit with a trustworthy pastoral professional. Or ask friends to recommend a member of the clergy whom you might visit. Most are well trained and willing to counsel men and women wrestling with health care decisions.

If you are not active in a faith community but desire spiritual guidance, consider calling your local hospital to see if there's a chaplain on staff. Hospital chaplains are delighted to assist you as you seek wisdom and comfort in the midst of a medical dilemma or crisis.

Round Out Your Spiritual Wheel

It is virtually impossible to become a highly healthy person without a balanced spiritual wheel. If your spiritual wheel is on the flat side—and up to this point in the book you've done nothing about it—now's the time. Make a decision today to talk to a friend or neighbor or colleague who seems to have a healthy and balanced spiritual wheel. If you don't know anyone like this, then call a member of the local clergy. Ask for an appointment to discuss your spiritual needs.

T = Take a Personal Inventory

Begin a personal inventory—in writing—about your health care needs. Buy a notebook or a small book with blank pages, and take some quiet time each day to think, meditate, pray, and journal. Don't just record the facts you're discovering. Record what others are telling you as well. What do trusted family members and friends have to say about your condition and the treatments you're considering? Also record how you feel about your medical, emotional, relational, and spiritual challenges. Stay honest. This journal is for no one's eyes but yours.

As part of your inventory, carefully consider what your own intuition is telling you about your medical problems. If you had no fear of any consequences, what would you do? If money were no object, what would you do? What do you sense God is leading you to do or not to do?

Write out your prayers, and spend plenty of time listening to the answers that come to you through your own spiritual ears, through the wise guidance of others, and through the circumstances that unfold. Record all answers that emerge from your time of prayer.

Finally, write about the support you feel you need, both now and throughout your treatment. What support is already available to you? How can you find the support you need?

Record Your Thoughts in Your Journal

Take five minutes every morning or evening to think about your personal inventory, any health care decisions with which you are struggling, or any steps you intend to take to improve your health. Write down all your thoughts in a brainstorming session. Don't hold anything back. Just write—for five minutes.

Then, at the end of two weeks, reread what you wrote down for each day. See if there's a pattern that may suggest a different approach or solution to something that's been bothering you.

Do this daily for a total of two weeks. Try not to miss a day.

MAKE A WELL-INFORMED DECISION

Following the G-U-E-S-T steps can help you make wise health care decisions—choices that are fully informed, spiritually sound, and personally satisfying. But remember, after all the learning and prayer and reflection, your final decision will involve a step of faith.

It's important to add a caveat here. My patients sometimes think that following this process somehow guarantees good results. It does not. All it can do is *improve* your chances for the best possible outcome.

Being informed about your options, expected outcomes, and any possible complications or side effects beforehand dramatically reduces the disappointment or anger that can arise from an undesirable outcome. Most disappointment and anger result from unmet expectations—disappointment if the expectation is lightly held, anger if the expectation is strongly held. Take, for example, a skin lesion removed from your face. Perhaps you expect no scar—that's an unrealistic expectation. Weeks later, however, there's still a faint scar, and you become angry or, at the very least, disappointed—emotions that generally aren't highly healthy.

When you become your own health care quarterback, you ask questions *before* any treatment is started. You learn about possible complications and side effects. You investigate the benefits of the treatment versus the problems it might create. There are no surprises. Your expectations are realistic.

Even so, if truth be told, there is no way in this imperfect world that you can ever be in complete control of the outcome. But if you have a healthy spiritual wheel, you can be assured that Someone is. According to the Bible, if we have a personal relationship with God, if we love him and live according to his plan and purposes, then in *all* things (good and bad) God will eventually work for our good. Even though we cannot be perfect health care quarterbacks, we can all choose to know the One who is.

Recheck Your Relationship with God

If by this point in the book you haven't begun a personal relationship with God, now might be the time to consider doing so. As the good health care quarterback you are—or might become—there's no wiser decision than to invite the One who created you and designed you, the One who knows the number of hairs on your head, into your life.

If you've never made that decision, turn back to page 124, where I describe how Wayne began his personal relationship with God. This is a decision you can make right now. You can not only ask your Creator to be on your team, but you can also, by a simple act of your will, become a member of *his* team.

USING THE TEMPLATE TO BECOME HIGHLY HEALTHY

The man with the foot inflammation (the plantar fasciitis), whose story I told earlier in this chapter, sent me an e-mail message a few months after his call to my radio show. Keith, who had been crippled for six months because of the pain from the inflammation, told me that after we talked he called his doctor's office for an appointment. He said he told the receptionist that he wasn't any better—in fact, his condition was worse. She was prepared to schedule a fifteen-minute appointment.

"No ma'am," he had replied, "I'm going to need a bit more time to talk this out with the doctor."

"But," she said, "our appointments are fifteen minutes."

He thought a second, then said, "Ma'am, can you please put me down for two appointments in a row?"

She did.

Keith went to the appointment, prepared with his questions, expecting to find the doctor not as helpful as he desired. He took his wife with him—knowing that the two of them were more likely to hear everything the doctor said.

Keith said he was surprised that the doctor entered the room with a sense of relief written all over his face and said, "Wow, how'd you get a thirty-minute appointment? That's a luxury for me! I'll have time to sit down."

This time, Keith said, the doctor took the time to get all the relevant facts about Keith's condition and medical history, then performed a thorough foot exam. He confirmed the diagnosis—plantar fasciitis—then listened to each of Keith's questions and explained several treatment options. The doctor recommended a referral to a foot surgeon but asked Keith if he needed time to consider this possibility—which he did.

Keith said he and his wife were delighted at how much they had learned during the visit. The nurse also gave them more information to study. At home Keith and his wife logged on to the Internet and read more about plantar fasciitis at several reputable medical sites. They asked two friends who had wrestled with the same problem about their experiences.

In the course of his research, Keith learned about a set of exercises that had recently been shown to help plantar fasciitis. He printed out the exercises (found on the Internet), along with an abstract of the accompanying article, and he took the information to his next appointment. Keith decided that, before considering surgery, he'd like to try several weeks of physical therapy and the home exercises.

Keith said the doctor gave him prescriptions for a new medication and for six weeks of physical therapy. He told Keith to wear his running shoes and do the exercises twice a day, then return in six weeks.

Keith said the doctor seemed as happy as he was to avoid surgery. "And he thanked me," Keith wrote. "Said I'd taught him a new trick that could help with other patients."

Keith had become his own health care quarterback and had learned how to team up with a winning health care team. Keith did it—and so can you!

CHAPTER TWELVE

Team Up with Winning Health Care Providers

The Essential of Teamwork

To be highly healthy requires not only that we choose to be our own health care quarterback (or have someone fill that role for us) but also that we choose positive associations with a health care coach (our primary personal physician) and other health care providers (our team players). Improving our health requires aligning ourselves with the best possible coach and players on a winning health care team.

Our Creator designed us to function best in cooperation with a team of people who love us and care for us. When this principle is combined with the principle of seeking wise advice and counsel from others, we have a strong foundation on which to build our winning health care team.

Once you've become convinced of the value of holistic health care—which embraces the physical, emotional, relational, and spiritual aspects of who you were created to be—then you can begin to build a winning health care team that shares, or at the very least is able to support, your beliefs and philosophy. Keeping these principles and caveats in mind, where can you find the best candidates for your team? How can you go about teaming up with health care

235

professionals and support persons who share a growing conviction that the ten essentials outlined in this book are critical to achieving high degrees of health?

WHO COULD BE ON YOUR WINNING HEALTH CARE TEAM?

Family and Friends

Before you began reading this book, I'm confident that you didn't even consider the possibility that family and friends could be—or should be—part of your health care team. Yet not only are they a part, they are a *crucial* part. Studies show that family and friends are consistently rated as the most vital supports for men and women who go through major health crises.

Nevertheless, as on any team, there can be harmful members. One of my most important roles as a family physician was helping to empower my patients to fire family members or friends who were negatively affecting their health and well-being—and who refused to change their attitudes or behavior. In his book *Don't Let Jerks Get the Best of You,* psychiatrist Paul Meier talks in great detail about how to do this—as does Jan Silvious in her book *Fool-Proofing Your Life.*

Too few team members can decrease the team's effectiveness as well. *But what if I have no family?* you may ask. *What if I've just moved to a new town and have no friends?* Then your assignment is to begin recruiting team members. I'm convinced that your health depends on it.

When I met Donald, he was in his late thirties and had just moved to our town to teach mathematics at the high school. He lived alone after divorcing several years earlier. He had no close friends, no hobbies, and no outside interests. He watched a lot of television.

He loved being a teacher, but his performance was being negatively affected by a variety of health problems. He came to me with symptoms of severe chronic pain along with sleep disturbance and low energy. His physical tests were all normal. His emotional tests showed no signs of depression or anxiety. His stress test was nearly normal. However, his relational and spiritual wheels were fairly flat. And he had never had a winning health care team to support him on his journey to becoming highly healthy.

On physical exam I found a plethora of what doctors call painful trigger points. My diagnosis was a then-not-well-known-and-still-difficult-to-treat disorder known as fibromyalgia syndrome (FMS). As I shared with Donald my diagnosis and prognosis, I also explained to him that I wouldn't be able to heal him. His forehead furrowed.

"Donald," I explained, "I can *help* you. But quite frankly, *you're* going to need to do a lot of the work of getting better. Are you willing?"

"Well, whatever it takes," Donald said. "It's got to be easier than living the way I'm living right now."

Besides my medical prescriptions, I gave Donald a prescription to find a small group of men with whom he could meet once a week for discussion and fellowship.

He thought for a second. "You know, I do know a principal at one of the elementary schools who is active in his church. He's also wrestling with some physical problems and has been through a divorce."

"He sounds like a good person to start with," I agreed. "Why not meet first with him, and then you guys can be on the lookout for others."

Within six months their group had grown to eight men. They met once a week for breakfast. They'd laugh; they'd study a passage of the Bible and pray for each other; they'd share from their hearts—and even cry. These guys grew to love each other, feel safe with each other, advise each other, and hold each other accountable to stay on the path toward health in all four wheels.

I watched Donald's health slowly improve. I'm convinced there is no way I could have ever done for Donald what this group of special friends did for him—and for each other. These men became a critical part of Donald's winning health care team.

Finding Friends

If you don't have at least one or two intimate friends, for the sake of your health, *now* is the time for you to seek them. Maybe you can begin building a close relationship with a colleague at work or school, with a family member who lives in town, or with someone you've met who has a similar hobby or interest.

Think through how you might build a relationship with this person. Take the initiative. If the person is open to a friendship, then begin to invest regular time in the relationship. Over time you'll be able to determine if the relationship is one in which you can safely share your life—your joys and your hurts and your medical challenges. Without this type of intimate relationship, you simply cannot be as healthy as you'd like to be.

Support Group

Having close relationships with at least a small number of friends or family members is just the opening round in creating a winning health care team.

If you're dealing with a particular health issue, then you'll also benefit from finding another kind of support group—an established group of folks who wrestle with the same health issues with which you struggle. You can usually locate such groups through local hospitals, national associations, or faith communities. Many physicians and mental health professionals provide information about such groups to their patients. Most medical centers and hospitals host groups like these. Such groups provide a great forum for the dissemination of useful information and the sharing of personal experience. They are also helpful to prevent or treat isolation, alienation, and loneliness.

These groups take a variety of forms. Some focus on a particular disease process (such as breast cancer and heart disease), others on addictions (alcohol, narcotics, sex, for example), and still others on emotional issues (such as depression, anxiety, and bipolar disease). These groups demonstrate the healing power of both sharing and listening. Even though the people in these groups start out as strangers, the "anonymous" setting in one sense makes it easier for some folks to open up and be vulnerable.

The Internet has transformed the meaning of the support group concept. On the Internet you can find hundreds of groups that are dealing with the same health issues and decisions you deal with. However, hear this: An Internet support group can never provide the same level of personal support and healing as a group of people with whom you meet face-to-face. Another warning: A number of studies have shown that the vast majority of the medical advice given in Internet chat rooms, bulletin boards, or support group Websites is inaccurate and sometimes even dangerous.

Donald, my patient with fibromyalgia, learned the hard way. He found a number of organizations on the Internet that kept him up-to-date on the worldwide research and developments regarding fibromyalgia. (Truth be told, much of what I know today about the syndrome and its treatment options I learned from Donald.) However, Donald made one mistake. He learned of a new dietary supplement recommended for fibromyalgia and ordered it over the Internet. He had been guaranteed that the substance was natural and safe and had no side effects. What he didn't know was that this supplement was likely to interact with both a prescription drug and another supplement he was taking. The unexpected interaction—causing a dramatic elevation in his blood pressure and heart rate—resulted in an ambulance ride to the emergency room. In this case, Donald's teammates who had told him about the dietary supplement thought they were helping him. Donald should have checked with the coach (me) before calling the play. But he didn't, and there was a flag on the play, and he was penalized. Thankfully, it was only a minor setback and didn't cost him the game!

Seek Support

If you decide to join a support group—or if you want to begin your own support group—then include only those who share these important goals: to be positive and truthful, to promote relational safety, to heal isolation, and to attend regularly.

Choose a facilitator who has good communication skills and who is committed to including each person in productive group discussion. Agree as a group that everything members share will remain strictly confidential. Commit yourself not only to sharing openly but also to listening carefully without a critical spirit. Focus on what you can contribute to the welfare of each person, while enjoying the positive results of receiving the kind of support and wise counsel that will help you become more highly healthy.

Mentor

If there is a lost art in America, it is the art of *mentoring.* The Bible encourages older and wiser men and women to guide the younger and less experienced—yet most who fit in this category don't follow this advice. I'm thankful for Bill Judge—a man who was a dairy farmer and the father of five girls, a man of common sense and uncommon wisdom. In 1985, I asked Bill if he would be my mentor. We met almost every Tuesday for nearly sixteen years. He would guide me, listen to me, pray for me, counsel me, advise me, teach me, and correct me. During those years, Barb and I faced scores of health decisions for ourselves and our children. I'm convinced that Bill's mentoring helped us become more highly healthy.

Master Mentoring

For more about mentoring, I recommend *As Iron Sharpens Iron,* a book written by Dr. Howard Hendricks and his son William. As you learn more about being mentored—or if you are older, about becoming a mentor—begin to pray and ask God to show you the person with whom you could have this kind of relationship. Once you sense who the person might be, call him or her and ask to meet for coffee or lunch. Propose your idea, and then give him or her time to think and pray about it. You'll find that having a mentor whose wisdom and guidance you trust can be an invaluable factor in becoming highly healthy.

Faith Community and Bible Study and Prayer Partners

Socialization is good for your health, but socialization in a worship or faith community is *exceptionally* good for your health. One of the keys to becoming highly healthy is to have people who will pray with you and for you. Increasingly, studies are showing that prayer affects a wide variety of health outcomes, including such issues as anxiety disorders, cardiovascular disease, depression, disabilities, marital satisfaction, pain relief, recovery from heart attack or an intensive care unit stay, recovery from surgery, substance abuse, and generalized well-being. Although not all studies have been able to demonstrate the effectiveness of prayer, those that have shown an effect have been impressive.

For example, one group of researchers demonstrated that the "strongest factors for well-being (life-satisfaction and happiness) were frequency of prayer and prayer experience." They also found that conversational and meditative prayers were more strongly related to well-being than was ritual or rote prayer.

In 1988, cardiologist Robert Byrd reported the results of a study in the coronary care unit at San Francisco General Hospital. The double-blind clinical trial involved almost 400 patients randomized to either an intercessory prayer group (a group that prayed for them) or a control group that did not receive prayer. Neither the doctors nor the patients knew who was being prayed for and who was not. In addition, the people praying did not know the patients for whom they were praying. The results were extraordinary: Patients in the prayer group had fewer bouts of heart failure, fewer cardiac arrests, and fewer pneumonias, and they used less medication and were less likely to be on a breathing machine.

Another prayer study found that rheumatoid arthritis patients who received in-person intercessory prayer (someone prayed for them in their presence) showed significant overall improvement over a one-year period. The researchers concluded, "In-person intercessory prayer may be a useful adjunct to standard medical care for certain patients with rheumatoid arthritis."

A study in South Korea compared two randomized groups of women going through in-vitro fertilization, looking at the conception rates of a group receiving intercessory prayer and a control group of patients who weren't prayed for. The researchers, who seemed stunned to find that the prayer group had a far higher pregnancy rate (50 percent, compared to 26 percent in the control group), concluded, "A statistically significant difference was observed for the effect of IP [intercessory prayer] on the outcome of IVF-ET [in vitro fertilization-embryo transfer]."

Practice Prayer and Bible Reading

If you are not a person of prayer, find someone who is. Ask this person if he or she will begin to pray for you and teach you to pray.

If you don't regularly read and study the Bible, now would be a good time to begin. Find a friend or pastor who studies the Bible and ask them to teach you how. Begin reading the Bible every day—even if for just a few minutes. Try to gradually increase your time. Ask a sales associate in your local bookstore to help you find a Bible that can provide guidance and interpretation as you read. You may want to look for a Bible that contains a "read the Bible in a year" plan, where each day's reading is organized in a way that highlights certain themes.

Both talking with God (prayer) and listening to God (Bible reading) increase your likelihood of becoming and remaining a highly healthy person.

Physicians and Physician Extenders

Obviously, a skillful physician is a critical part of any health care team. I highly recommend that you choose a primary care physician (PCP)—a health care coach—and begin to build a trusting relationship with him or her. Your PCP will serve as your generalist, managing your overall care and working closely with you to make most of the medical decisions you face. In many health insurance plans, care by specialists is paid for only if your PCP refers you. Primary care represents the most basic level of the American health care system.

The value of a PCP is in having someone who knows you and who can collaborate with other providers, when necessary, in identifying and addressing your individual comprehensive health care needs. Having a PCP allows you to establish a trusting relationship with a physician over time, maintain continuity in your personal health care, and move easily between crisis-oriented (acute) health care problems and preventive care and health maintenance.

In addition, many people are seeing the value of what are called midlevel providers, or physician extenders—highly trained physician assistants (PA), certified nurse midwives (CNM), and nurse practitioners (NP). PAs and NPs usually work with a physician and often have more time to devote to your care than the doctor has. NPs (in some jurisdictions) and CNMs (in most locales) can also work independently of a physician. Services provided by midlevel providers cost less.

A 1986 study conducted by the Congressional Office of Technology Assessment concluded that care provided by nurse practitioners, physician assistants, and certified nurse midwives (within their respective areas of expertise) was equivalent to the care provided by physicians for the same conditions. The study reported that NPs and CNMs were found to be more adept than physicians in some areas of preventive care and patient communication, while PAs were reported to be more adept than physicians in some areas of supportive care and health promotion. In addition, NPs, PAs, and CNMs all consult with or refer to physicians as needed for problems encountered that are outside their scopes of practice.

Although some physicians find such studies offensive, many more are learning how to work effectively with these very skilled men and women. It would only be fair to point out that this study compared midlevel providers with all physicians. My guess is that primary care physicians would have fared much better than many of their colleagues in these areas.

Mental Health Professionals

Psychologists, professional counselors, social workers, and marriage and family therapists are licensed, certified, and trained to provide diagnosis and therapy for a variety of mental, emotional, and relational problems. They do not prescribe medication. They often work in conjunction with your personal physician.

Pastoral counselors and chaplains can help with spiritual problems, as well as with some emotional and relational problems, but for more severe emotional or relational issues I usually recommend seeing a licensed mental health therapist in one of the mental health disciplines mentioned above.

Psychiatrists can also play an important role on your health care team. Psychiatrists are M.D.s who are specially trained in evaluating and treating mental health and disease. They prescribe medications, order laboratory and other diagnostic tests, and admit patients to the hospital. Psychiatrists usually work in tandem with a team of mental health professionals.

A counseling program to which I've frequently referred my patients is the Meier New Life Clinics. In addition, you can call the counseling department at Focus on the Family (1-800-A-FAMILY) to obtain the names of competent faith-based counselors in your area.

One of the healthy habits that my wife, Barb, and I have practiced for years is to visit a mental health professional annually—together. Our goal is to have the professional check our emotional and relational wheels.

One year, the counselor asked Barb a question. I thought I knew the answer. You can imagine my surprise when she answered exactly opposite from what I expected. I was stunned. It was something I could have easily addressed if she had simply told me.

"Honey," I protested, "why didn't you tell me?"

She looked at me so innocently and replied, "Well, *you* didn't ask me. *He* did."

'Nuf said!

Pastoral or Psychological Preventive Care

Would a visit to a psychologist or pastoral counselor every year or two be wise for you and your family (if you have a family)? Consider such a checkup as a preventive medicine exam for your emotional, relational, and spiritual wheels. If you do decide to go, keep an open attitude, expecting to find additional areas in which you can improve and become more highly healthy.

Registered Dietitians

Registered dietitians are an invaluable source for physicians and patients alike regarding nutrition and dietary management of a host of conditions. Many have private practices; others serve on the staff of local hospitals and are available for private consultations. They are licensed by the state.

You've probably discovered that the average physician has little or no training in nutrition. And you know from reading this book that your nutrition affects your physical, emotional, and relational health wheels. If you think your or your family's nutritional habits are in need of repair, ask your doctor to refer you to a dietitian for a consultation. He or she will take a careful diet history and then will be able to suggest healthy strategies for improving your nutritional health. It could well be one of the best hours of consultation you'll ever spend.

Consider the Roflinger family. Bill, Sherry, and their four kids were all overweight, and several of them were experiencing health difficulties as a result. They resisted my suggestion to make some changes in this area of their health until Bill's dad died of a heart attack at the age of fifty-eight. *Now* they were interested. The funeral was a traumatic time for them all.

Our hospital dietitians offered a weekly nutrition class for local residents. I suggested that the Roflingers commit to attending these classes for three months—and they did. They learned how to cook their favorite meals in healthier ways. They learned how to dine *together* and gain great benefit for their family life. They learned about portion control, good versus bad sugars, and good versus bad fats. They learned how to eat in a healthier fashion. They even learned how to exercise as a family.

I wish you could have seen them one year later. They were all approaching their ideal body weight. Bill was no longer taking blood pressure medication. Sherry was off her diabetes medication. The kids were looking good and feeling good. The entire family was getting positive feedback from family and friends.

Clergy or Pastoral Professionals

A wise addition to a person's health care team is a spiritual adviser. Pastors, priests, rabbis, and other spiritual professionals such as chaplains and pastoral counselors are obvious selections. In many faith communities, elders, deacons, or specially trained lay leaders also can fill this role. Of note are those trained by the Order of St. Luke and the Stephen Ministry. Both of these ministries train laypeople to minister to the health needs of others. If you want to learn more, you can access their information via my Website at www.highlyhealthy.net.

Chiropractors

Many people choose to have a chiropractor on their health care team. A chiropractor is a health care provider who utilizes musculoskeletal therapies such as manipulation, stretching, and other physical therapies. Many chiropractors believe that disease is caused by misalignments of the spine—what they call *subluxations*—that pinch the nerves going from the spinal column to the body. They believe that after proper manipulations or adjustments, normal nerve transmissions are restored and the body can resume its innate ability to recover from illness—or even to prevent illness.

From my viewpoint—and that of the overwhelming majority of scientists—there is virtually no scientific evidence to support the subluxation theory. Author Stephen Barrett, M.D., points out that the definition of *subluxation* is "incomplete or partial dislocation—a condition, visible on x-ray films, in which the bony surfaces of a joint no longer face each other exactly but remain partially aligned." Dr. Barrett declares, "No such condition can be corrected by chiropractic treatment." He goes on to note, "Chiropractors also differ about how to find 'subluxations' and where they are located. In addition to seeing them on x-ray films, chiropractors say they can find them by: (a) feeling the spine with their hand, (b) measuring skin temperature near the spine with an instrument, (c) concluding that one of the patient's legs is 'functionally' longer than the other, (d) studying the shadows produced by a device that projects a beam of light onto the patient's back, (e) weighing the patient on special scales, and/or (f) detecting 'nerve irritation' with a device. Undercover investigations in which many chiropractors have examined the same patient have found that the diagnoses and proposed treatments differed greatly from one practitioner to another."

Over the years, chiropractic care has slowly separated into two camps: the *traditional chiropractors,* who adhere strictly to the original philosophy of only locating and eliminating subluxations, and the *modern chiropractors,* who combine musculoskeletal manipulation and adjustments with other adjunct therapies such as gentle stretching, trigger-point treatments, hot or cold treatments, nutrition counseling and therapies, supplement recommendations, and exercise programs.

The majority of practicing chiropractors today fall into the modern category, frequently using new technologies to locate and eliminate subluxations. However, there's a split in this camp, too. Among the modern chiropractors are two primary schools of thought: (1) the *isolationists,* who believe their therapy can prevent and treat most diseases without the assistance of other health care providers (they prefer to work in isolation and often have a disdain for anyone in the traditional medical world), and (2) the science-based *rationalists,* who desire to be part of a traditional health care team.

It is surely possible for chiropractors who are team players to play a valuable role on your health care team when needed. Samuel Homola, D.C., writes the following:

> Spinal manipulation can relieve some types of back and neck pain and other conditions related to tightness and loss of mobility, such as tension headache or aching in muscles and joints. We also know that massage may be as effective as cervical manipulation in relieving tension headache. And physical therapy techniques may be as effective as spinal manipulation in long-term relief of back pain. Rational chiropractors can offer all of these modalities, when appropriate, and thus provide patients with a choice. . . .
>
> Science-based chiropractors make appropriate judgments about the nature of their patients' problems, determine whether these problems lie within their scope, and make appropriate referrals for problems that do not. If you can find one who uses manipulation and physical therapy appropriately and who is willing to coordinate with your personal physician, you can benefit from the best that both have to offer.

I agree with Dr. Homola. For years, my practice consulted a modern, rational, science-based chiropractor—to my and my patients' benefit. The patients most helped by this type of chiropractic care had acute musculo-skeletal injuries—especially some forms of neck and back pain. I recommend that you *don't* use a chiropractor as your primary care physician, but only when needed.

The licensing of chiropractors differs significantly from state to state. Currently the majority of states require successful completion of the National Chiropractic Board examination prior to licensure. Some states also require passing a practical examination in addition to the written board exam.

Alternative Health Care Providers

More and more Americans are asking alternative, or complementary, health care providers to be members of their health care team. Many of these alternative practitioners are unlicensed and unregulated, particularly those who deal in alternative nutritional therapy.

In *Alternative Medicine,* you can read about what Dónal O'Mathúna and I discovered as we researched the most popular alternative therapies, herbal remedies, vitamins, and dietary supplements available in today's health market-place. We looked at the forty-or-so most purchased alternative therapies used in the United States—everything from acupuncture to yoga—and about sixty of the most purchased herbs, vitamins, and supplements—everything from aloe to zinc.

We not only looked at what people said they did, we also looked at the evidence, if any, to support each therapy for each disease or condition it was supposed to treat. We also examined any underlying spiritual issues that might affect a patient's decision to use or avoid a particular therapy.

We found several alternatives to traditional care that have evidence to support their use—and even more alternatives with good evidence that they could complement traditional medicine. However, we also found that most alternative therapies had little or no evidence to back up their claims, and we found many we considered to be downright dangerous. We concluded that if you choose to add alternative therapies to your health care, or if you seek the services of an alternative practitioner, be sure to do so under the supervision of your health care coach—your primary care physician.

HOW TO HIRE A HEALTH CARE PROVIDER

There are several important steps to take in hiring the health care providers for your winning health care team. Ask others for referrals and recommendations. You'll want to determine if a particular provider's personality and philosophy of care match your desires. Check the provider's qualifications and track record, and schedule an interview—to see if you and the provider will work well together on your journey to becoming highly healthy.

Find a Good Fit

Choosing the best physician for yourself or for a loved one requires some information gathering. While many insurance companies limit your choices to physicians they have approved, you should still decide the following:

- Do you want a physician who is disease oriented or wellness oriented?
- Do you prefer conservative or aggressive approaches to care?
- Would you rather have a physician who is informal and warm, or formal and detached?
- What specific competencies do you want in your physician? Pediatric care? Maternity care? Hospital care? Care for the entire family? Elder care? Care for a specific disease or condition?
- Do you prefer a physician who invites your participation in your care or one who tells you what to do?
- Do you desire a male or a female physician?
- Do you want a physician who is interested in or at least supportive of your spiritual interests?

Get Referrals and Recommendations

Once you've determined your personal preferences, begin to ask friends, neighbors, colleagues, relatives, or clergy for names of doctors they'd recommend. Check especially with trustworthy people who are connected in some way to the health care system. Always consider the opinion of other reliable providers who have cared for you in the past. If you have specialized needs for a specific physical or mental problem, local and state advocate or support groups can be an excellent source of information about providers who are skilled in these areas.

To further narrow your search, consider checking to see if public information about the prospective provider is available. Sources of such information include the appropriate state professional organization, the Better Business Bureau, and your state's department of professional regulation and insurance. Some states also have Internet databases that allow you to gather information about malpractice cases and complaints. The state should be able to tell you if the physician is currently licensed and if the state has ever taken disciplinary action against him or her. In most states you may request a copy of the disciplinary order.

To find out if any malpractice lawsuits have been filed against a physician, in most states you can check with the county where the physician practices and resides. This list is usually maintained in the county clerk's office. Keep in mind, however, that anyone can file a lawsuit at any time and for just about any reason. The existence of a malpractice complaint or lawsuit doesn't automatically suggest that a physician is a bad doctor. It may only mean that one particular patient was unhappy about something. What's more, the outcome may have been out of the physician's control. However, several legal actions, or a pattern of similar actions, may be cause for concern.

There are several Internet databases that will inform you of a potential physician's record—including the American Medical Association's "AMA Physician Select" Website, which you can access via www.highlyhealthy.net. The AMA says this site provides information on virtually every licensed physician in the United States and its possessions.

Once you've determined the doctors who make it to the top of your list, call their offices. Ask the receptionist if a staff member can take a few moments to answer these questions:

- Are you accepting new patients?
- Do you accept my insurance plan?
- How long has the doctor practiced in this area?
- How many patients are seen by this practice?
- Does the doctor practice alone or in a group? If in a group, how many members are there and how many offices do they practice in?
- Who provides my care when the doctor is not available?
- At which hospitals does the doctor admit patients, and are there any limitations on the doctor's hospital privileges?
- If the doctor does not admit patients, who will care for me if I have to go to the emergency room or have to be admitted to the hospital?
- Is the doctor certified by a medical specialty board? Which board? In what specialty area?
- If I call with a question or problem, will the doctor speak to me personally? When is the best time to call?
- How often does the doctor recommend routine physicals? Will they be covered by my health plan? What does the doctor routinely check for, and what tests are generally done?
- Can a friend or family member sit in on my exams and procedures?
- How willing is the doctor to have me take an active role in my treatment? How would he or she react if I asked about a medication or test

that he or she wasn't familiar with or if I brought in my own informal research for review with the doctor?
- How does the doctor feel about alternative medicine?

Schedule an Interview

Once you choose a particular health care provider, request a brief appointment to interview him or her. More and more providers welcome these interviews, and they allow you to ask specific questions related to the expectations you have for the coordination and management of your personal health care. Increasingly, providers offer this type of appointment at no cost to you. After you leave the interview, ask yourself these questions:

- Was I treated courteously and respectfully?
- Was the office orderly, comfortable, and clean?
- Was the staff friendly and helpful?
- Did I have to wait a long time past my appointment time to see the doctor?
- Were all of my questions answered?
- Did I feel rushed or disrespected or disregarded?

If you were not satisfied, go to the next name on your list!

You may want to check out a couple of resources that give you additional information on picking a doctor. *Examining Your Doctor* by Timothy McCall, M.D., puts the white coat on *you,* and the horrid paper gown—which is open down the back—on your physician and hospital. There is a very helpful article on choosing the right doctor for your needs, which you can access via my Website at www.highlyhealthy.net.

Practice an Attitude of Gratitude with Your Physician

If you already have a winning health care team and don't need to find new players, why not consider jotting a brief thank-you note to your health care provider, physician, or other member of your team. So many of them hear only complaints. Rare is the appreciative patient who will write and just say, "You are doing a great job, and I appreciate you so much."

If you feel this way, write or e-mail a note to your doctor or provider today.

Take a Spiritual Inventory

Finding a doctor and other health care team members who share your spiritual foundation and practices may be crucial for you—and thankfully it's fairly simple. You can use a *spiritual inventory.*

Doctors are increasingly using spiritual inventories in their care of patients. In fact, when I make presentations at medical centers, medical schools, and professional meetings, the question I most often hear is, How can doctors take useful spiritual inventories of their patients?

In the same way a doctor can inquire about a patient's spiritual beliefs, a patient should feel free to ask about how a doctor's spiritual beliefs and practices relate to his or her medical care. A winning health care provider should be perfectly willing to let you know where he or she stands on these issues. Furthermore, when it comes to alternative or complementary care providers, these questions can be critical, because some have been known to use their therapy to actively recruit unsuspecting patients into spiritual belief systems I think are highly unhealthy.

Here are a few questions you could ask at your interview of the prospective health care provider—or during your first official appointment. I'm sure you could come up with some of your own to add. I'm aware that most people probably won't follow my suggestion to ask a provider *all* the following questions—especially at a first meeting. However, if your spirituality is very important to you, and if you want a provider who shares your beliefs, then each question might by useful for you to discuss with your physician at some point.

1. Are you willing to consider my spiritual preferences as you care for me?
2. Are you open to discussion of the religious or spiritual implications of my health care?
3. Are you willing to work with my spiritual mentors (pastor, priest, rabbi, elder) and other members of my health care team (family, friends, mentor, support group) in providing me with the best possible health care?
4. Are you willing to pray with me—or for me—if I feel the need for prayer?

For those who are working to inflate and balance their spiritual wheel, asking questions 1, 2, 3, and 4 is perfectly reasonable—and, I would expect, acceptable to most physicians and providers. Some might consider the following questions 5 through 9 to be too personal and intimate to ask of a total stranger. So if you're not there—no problem.

5. What does spirituality mean to you? How much is religion (and God) a source of strength and comfort for you?

6. Have you ever had an experience that convinced you that God or a higher power exists?

7. How strongly religious or spiritually oriented do you consider yourself to be?

8. Do you pray? If so, how frequently?

9. Do you attend religious worship times? If so, how often do you generally attend?

Even if you decide that asking these questions in an interview style is not comfortable, you may want to look for opportunities to talk informally during a visit. But at least consider asking the first four questions. Frankly discussing this can strengthen all four of your health wheels, as well as your trust relationship with your health care provider.

HOW TO WORK EFFECTIVELY WITH A HEALTH CARE GIVER

To work effectively with your health care team requires effort on both your part and their part. The doctor-patient relationship operates best and most effectively when both parties are working together. In other words, as a patient you have both rights and responsibilities. Let's look first at your rights. You have the right to . . .

- choose your doctor. Some insurance companies and HMOs make it difficult, but you can usually choose a health plan that lets you choose a physician. In his new book *Power to the Patient,* Dr. Isadore Rosenfeld says that finding a physician with whom you are compatible is nearly as important as selecting your spouse. (I suspect he's using hyperbole, but it *is* an important decision.)

- know of any and all financial relationships between your doctors, your insurance company, and your hospital. For example, if your doctor is hired by your employer or your insurance company, then your doctor is legally and ethically bound to care, first and foremost, for the needs of the "company." You want to be sure that your doctor is working for you and seeking, first and foremost, *your* well-being.

- receive courteous, considerate, and civil care—to be treated with respect and dignity. If your doctor or the doctor's staff is frequently rude or discourteous, then you have every right to fire them.

- receive preventive care (in each of the four health wheels) as well as acute care.

- be seen within a reasonable time for a scheduled appointment—or to be informed of any delays and given the option to see another provider or professional, reschedule your appointment, or continue waiting. Any prolonged wait should occur only with your consent.
- receive medical care that meets or exceeds the national standards of acceptable care.
- receive impartial access to high-quality, cost-effective, and evidence-based medical treatment regardless of race, sex, religion, or national origin.
- receive medical care that takes into account the social, emotional, relational, cultural, and spiritual beliefs and practices that affect your feelings about disease or treatment—as long as your belief does not cause someone else to violate his or her conscience.
- be guaranteed of reasonable safety, comfort, and privacy within medical facilities.
- be protected from preventable harm during treatments or procedures.
- not be treated by health care providers or professionals who are sleep deprived, under undue mental duress, or under the influence of drugs or alcohol.
- be protected from individuals who might harm you or cause an unnatural death of either you, your loved one, or your unborn child.
- be fully informed by your primary care physician about your diagnosis (or the list of other diagnoses the doctor is looking to rule out), condition, treatment, and prognosis.
- be fully informed of your medical options and their significant complications, risks, benefits, and costs.
- be fully informed of the doctor's or hospital's track record for any recommended surgery or procedure—note that typically you must ask for this information.
- know the cost of any and all proposed treatments before they are rendered.
- be fully informed of any available alternative treatments and any additional information required for your fully informed consent before any treatment or procedure.
- gain a second (or third or fourth) opinion about your medical condition or proposed treatment options.
- read and understand your medical records at a time that is mutually convenient for you and your health care team. (Not all physicians agree, but if this is important to you, be sure to seek a physician who will support this.)
- have the information in your medical record explained to you.

- expect that any discussion or consultation involving your care will be conducted in the strictest confidence.
- expect privacy and confidentiality of your medical records.
- have your health records read only by individuals who are involved in your treatment, care, or the monitoring of its quality.
- receive continuity of care.
- be told if your care or treatment is in any way experimental.
- have an impartial appeal process and an objective, rapid review of any claims or requests for treatments denied by your insurance company.
- refuse any treatment or care you do not desire and to be informed of the consequences of your decision.

With all these rights, of course, come responsibilities. In fact, in my opinion, rights can only be conferred in an environment in which responsibilities are taken seriously. Here are just a few of your responsibilities if you want to be in a highly healthy doctor-patient relationship. You are responsible to . . .

- be sure the office staff understands your needs and expectations as you schedule appointments—so they can help make sure you have enough time scheduled for your needs.
- keep your appointments. If for any reason you cannot keep an appointment, you are responsible to notify your doctor in a timely manner.
- provide accurate and complete information about your current complaints; past illnesses and hospitalizations; other past medical history; current medications (including herbs, vitamins, and supplements); any allergic reactions to medications; family and social history (including sexual history); recent changes in your condition; and any other significant conditions related to your physical, emotional, relational, or spiritual health.
- have your medical records transferred to your new physician's office. Only you can authorize the release of your records, and you'll have to sign a release to do so.
- make it known to your health care provider whenever you do not understand *any* part of a recommended course of action or expectation made of you during this course of action.
- ask questions if you're confused and don't understand something about your care, treatment, or medications.
- follow the instructions and prescribed treatment plan(s) recommended by your health care professional—unless you clearly indicate the reasons you cannot or will not.
- live with the consequences of any of your actions if you refuse treatment or don't follow a health care team member's instructions.

- respond to your health care team in a respectful and courteous manner.
- be considerate of the rights of other patients and health care personnel.
- find care for your children during your medical treatment or appointment—unless your health care team agrees to provide child care during your appointment.
- not bring additional children along for a child's medical treatment or appointment—unless your health care team agrees to provide child care during your child's appointment.
- help your health care team accurately maintain a complete medical record.
- double-check all medications prescribed or administered to you at any time, especially being aware of any allergic reactions.
- hire (or fire) the health care team of your choosing—note, though, that your choice may not be covered by your health insurance contracts.

Review Your Rights and Responsibilities

Carefully review the lists of your rights and your responsibilities. Delete those that aren't important to you—or those with which you disagree.

Next time you see a member of your health care team (or the next time you interview a person for your team), ask them if they are willing to attempt to meet this standard of winning care. If they refuse, you may want to find someone who *will* agree to care for you the way you need to be cared for.

HOW TO FIRE A HEALTH CARE GIVER

Remember Keith? He was astounded at my suggestion that he could—and should—fire any doctor or health care provider who refused to work with him in an effective way. He had figured out what he wanted from his health care providers, and he was learning how to ask for what was appropriate—for what he deserved. Still, the thought that he had the option—and the obligation—to replace members of his health care team who weren't pulling their weight was rather unsettling. Because most people have been taught that "doctor knows best" or "the doctor is the boss," they may not have thought much about how to terminate the relationship with health care providers who don't provide good care.

One of my friends recently had just such an opportunity. Jill has been following many of my prescriptions—particularly those related to being her own health care quarterback and teaming up with winning health care providers. Having suffered from chronic lower back pain for almost a decade, this relatively young woman had had enough. She scheduled an appointment with her primary care physician to discuss her pain and to get professional guidance on how to cope better—or, far better, eliminate the pain altogether.

Jill's primary care physician, a caring and patient woman with a small private practice, talked with my friend at length and examined her carefully. The doctor could see no obvious reason for her patient's high level of pain, so she wisely recommended that Jill get an MRI (magnetic resonance imaging) scan to aid in the diagnostic process.

The doctor's nurse checked with Jill's insurance company to make sure that this expensive procedure would be covered. Then the nurse found the local laboratory that could provide the procedure under Jill's health plan. With the lab's phone number in hand, Jill was able to schedule an appointment within a week.

Once the results were available, the lab sent a report to Jill's doctor, and the two of them met to talk. Jill's doctor explained in detail—with the help of a visual aid (a rubber skeleton that showed all the parts of the human spine and the connecting muscles and ligaments)—precisely what appeared to be causing Jill's back pain. A skiing accident nearly fifteen years earlier had likely been the culprit, causing an injury to two of Jill's disks, which in turn began to affect the surrounding tissues and produce the chronic pain in her lower back.

So far, so good: Some bad news, but at least a diagnosis and a thorough explanation. Jill had the facts about what was wrong with her. Now she wanted to find out whether there was anything she could do about it.

Her doctor gave Jill the name of a well-respected surgeon and suggested that she make an appointment to discuss her condition and his recommendations. Jill immediately looked alarmed. The doctor reassured her that there often were other options besides surgery, and she might not be a good candidate for it anyway. Jill's doctor also referred her to a chronic pain specialist who could help her determine her best course of treatment for managing the pain from her injury.

Jill was on a roll. She promptly made an appointment with the pain specialist and showed up with a list of a dozen or so excellent questions designed to prompt productive discussion about treatment options. She was excited to finally be getting somewhere! She could almost feel her back pain subsiding as she worked to hook up with the right team members who could educate and guide her.

You can imagine her disappointment when she met her new doctor and found him to be not only hurried (she had asked his nurse to schedule her for a full thirty minutes) but also brusque, cold, and contemptuous of Jill's careful preparation for the appointment. Rather than congratulate her on being a great quarterback, he shamed her for daring to ask so many basic questions (which Jill said he seemed to think were stupid and beneath him). He repeatedly looked at his watch and at his shoes (not at his patient), while Jill tried to engage him in a productive discussion of her health care concerns. He gave very brief answers to her questions and made it plain that she wasn't welcome to ask for any clarification or expansion.

Then, before even ten minutes had passed, he abruptly stood up, told Jill he was too busy to continue what he clearly didn't think was his job—to educate his patient—and handed her the card of a physical therapist he said he would recommend. Without so much as a handshake, he bolted from the room.

As Jill dressed and gathered her list of questions and the MRI films (the "expert" wouldn't even look at these), she felt absolutely deflated. In fact, she felt ashamed. *I guess I was just way out of line,* she told herself. *I was stupid to get so excited about maybe getting some answers and some relief from this pain after all these years.* Jill told me she literally broke into tears once she got to her car. She felt humiliated and hopeless.

Fortunately, Jill isn't the type of person to give up easily. The next day she called the physical therapist. She had no idea why the pain specialist recommended physical therapy or what she might expect in terms of treatment. But she made an appointment and, with the same list of questions in hand, went to see the physical therapist the following week.

Well, not only was the therapist "the answer to my prayers," Jill told me, but he also worked hard with Jill (and her insurance company) over a three-month period. He enthusiastically answered every question and gave her information she hadn't even thought to ask for. He put together a customized exercise plan that specifically addressed Jill's source of pain. He treated her like the intelligent woman she is, and he even made her painful therapy fun! Now, nearly five months after completing therapy and learning a host of spine-stabilizing and muscle-strengthening exercises—none of which require expensive machines or detailed instructions—Jill is highly motivated to continue her exercise program indefinitely at home.

"Walt," she told me recently, "I'm absolutely amazed at the difference in my body. Before treatment I'd been feeling as though I was out of the race at only forty years of age. I was starting to feel practically disabled, even though I'm very healthy in most other areas. I can't tell you what a relief it is to discover that by doing these exercises daily, I can not only make a huge difference in my pain level, which has dropped dramatically, but also in my overall sense of well-being. I feel stronger physically, more hopeful emotionally, and—perhaps most important—empowered as my own health care quarterback. I *could* get the health care I needed—and I did!"

Jill's final step was to officially fire Dr. Zero. He had insisted—while rushing out of the examining room—that she make a follow-up appointment in three weeks. She had felt intimidated enough to follow his orders. But after only one session with her physical therapist, Jill knew she'd never go back for "care" from this uncaring physician. She phoned his office and canceled her appointment. She asked the receptionist to thank him for recommending the fine physical therapist. And then she dropped a note in the mail, informing the doctor that she would never be back—and why. Politely and succinctly, she explained that she *would* not be treated with such disrespect and that she was very disappointed in the lack of care she received from this specialist. She never heard back from him.

"Walt," she told me, "now all the players on my health care team are people I trust and respect—who give me the care I want and deserve. As uncomfortable as this experience was for me, it taught me a lot. I've taken the right steps to deal with my condition, and I feel younger than I have in years!"

All I could think of when Jill was telling me this was, *You did it! You did it!*

Evaluate Your Health Care Team

As you've evaluated your health care team, would you rate all team members as winners? If not, which team members do you need to replace?

Remember, these team members are, for the most part, supposed to serve you. And most are paid quite well to do so. If you need to make any changes, *now* is the time to think through how and when this might best be accomplished. Begin your search for replacements today!

CONCLUSION

Congratulations! You've done it!

By reading this entire book, you've traveled down a road few people take—a pathway toward understanding the essentials of becoming a highly healthy person. And this is a great start! However, reading this book and beginning to apply some of its principles are only the beginning steps. Now you must make a very important decision—one that may well affect the quality and length of your life.

This decision is predicated on the fact that virtually no person will be able to apply all the principles in this book in a few days or weeks. Let me say it more bluntly and clearly: It can't be done! You can't do it in eight days or eight weeks—but you don't have to. I suspect it would take the average person a year or more to apply most of these decisions on a consistent basis.

Here's your homework:

Set Some Goals

In your journal, select a page and make two columns. Over the left column write, **Things I've Done or Am Doing**. Over the right column write, **Things I Need to Do**.

Take time to read back through each of the assessments you've completed. Look also at your journal entries and review the prescriptions in each chapter. Then carefully consider what you've accomplished and where you've fallen short. Enter each item in one column or the other.

Then spend time looking through the left column. What still needs improvement and how and when can you work on these things? Make notes to yourself.

Now turn your attention to the right column. Number the items. Prioritize them in this order: Begin with the item that would be the easiest to accomplish. The last number should be given to the task that will be the most difficult.

Go through the list again and be sure that you make your goals and plans as specific as possible. The more specific you are about your destination, the more likely you are to arrive. Now pick a date by which you want to accomplish each goal. Be sure to give yourself plenty of time to accomplish each one. Accomplishing the goals—even if done slowly—is much more important than setting goals you can't reach. Write next to the item the date when you expect to accomplish each goal.

Remember that you are a work in progress. Relax and use your goals and plans to discover and reinforce what is important to you and what is important in life.

Recruit Assistance and Accountability

Over the next few weeks, review these goals with members of your health care team—keeping two things in mind:

- Have your teammates review the appropriateness of your goals, priorities, and timetable. If they don't seem appropriate, adjust them!
- Ask your teammates which goals they'd be willing to help you with.

With accountability and assistance, you're much more likely to become a highly healthy person.

Have Fun!

You're already on your way to becoming highly healthy. So relax and plan to have fun. Just starting down this road is a tremendous accomplishment.

As you look back through your goals and plans, look for the ones that would be the most fun for you to carry out. Go ahead—move them to the top of your list! The more fun you have working toward your health goals, the more likely you are to become highly healthy.

Here's another tip: Look for ways you can combine goals and plans. For example, if you stop smoking, save the money you used to spend on cigarettes and treat yourself to a vacation six months later. If you lose weight, treat yourself by purchasing some new clothing.

The bottom line: Enjoy the process! Choosing legitimate plans and goals that are fun can be a great motivator.

Don't Become Discouraged!

If you follow these steps, then most of your goals will be reachable. But don't worry if you miss one or more. Even if you achieve only half of your goals, you'll be well down the road to becoming more highly healthy.

Don't let yourself get discouraged. If you can't meet a goal, talk it over with one of the members of your health care team—and then reset your goal. Over time, you can reach them all—one at a time.

Before you close the book, I want to thank you for allowing me to spend this precious time with you. The opportunity you've given me to work with you on becoming a more highly healthy person has been an honor and a privilege.

1. When a teenager drives by my yard with the car stereo blaring acid rock, I can feel my blood pressure starting to rise.   T   F

2. There are several people whom I trust to help solve my problems.   T   F

3. During the past week, I was bothered on three or more days by things that usually don't bother me.   T   F

4. If my haircutter were to trim off more hair than I wanted, I'd let him or her know in no uncertain terms.   T   F

5. If I needed help fixing an appliance or repairing my car, there is someone who could help me.   T   F

6. When I'm in the express "twelve items only" line at the supermarket, I almost always glance ahead to see if anyone has more than twelve items.   T   F

7. Most of my friends are more interesting than I am.   T   F

8. During the past week, on three or more days I did not feel like eating; my appetite was poor.   T   F

9. At work the pace is usually very hectic.   T   F

10. Most homeless people in large cities are down-and-out because they lack ambition or self-discipline.   T   F

11. There is someone who takes pride in my accomplishments.   T   F

12. At times in the past when I was very angry with someone, I have on occasion hit or shoved that person.   T   F

13. When I feel lonely, there are several people I can talk to.   T   F

     T   F

14. During the past week, there were three or more   T   F
    days when I felt that I could not shake off the
    blues, even with help from my family or friends.

15. When I read in the news about drug-related
    crime, I wish the government had better educa-   T   F
    tional and drug detoxification programs, even
    for pushers.   T   F

16. There is no one I feel comfortable talking to
    about intimate personal problems.

17. The AIDS epidemic is largely the result of irre-   T   F
    sponsible behavior on the part of a small pro-
    portion of the population.   T   F

18. During the past week I felt that I was just as
    good as other people more than half the time.   T   F

19. Apart from work, the pace of my life is very
    hectic.   T   F

20. When arguing with a friend or relative, I find   T   F
    profanity an effective tool.

21. I often meet or talk with family or friends.   T   F

22. When stuck in a traffic jam, I quickly become   T   F
    irritated and annoyed.

23. Most people I know think highly of me.   T   F

24. When a really important job needs to be done,
    I prefer to do it myself.

25. If I needed a ride to the airport very early in the   T   F
    morning, I would have a hard time finding
    someone to take me.

26. During the past week, there were three or more   T   F
    days when I had trouble keeping my mind on   T   F
    what I was doing.

27. My work is very demanding.   T   F

28. I usually prefer to keep my angry feelings to
    myself.   T   F

29. I feel as though my circle of friends doesn't
    always include me.   T   F

30. If another driver butts ahead of me in traffic, I'll
    drop back to avoid him or her.   T   F

31. There really is no one who can give me an objective view of how I'm handling my problems. T F
32. I felt depressed on three or more days during the past week. T F
33. If someone treats me unfairly, I'm apt to keep thinking about it for hours. T F
34. There are several different people I enjoy spending time with.
35. When the cars ahead of me on an unfamiliar road start to slow down and stop as they approach a curve, I usually assume someone up ahead has had a fender bender or worse. T F

T F

36. I think that my friends feel I'm not very good at helping them solve their problems. T F
37. During the past week, there were three or more days when I felt that everything I did was an effort. T F
38. I'll usually try to correct another person who expresses an ignorant belief. T F

T F

39. I experience being at home or engaging in leisure activities as very demanding. T F
40. It doesn't bother me to be in slow-moving bank or supermarket lines. T F
41. If I was sick and needed a friend, family member, or acquaintance to take me to the doctor, I would have trouble finding someone. T F
42. When someone is being rude or annoying, I can get rough with him or her. T F
43. If I wanted to go on a trip for a day (for example, to the beach), I would have a hard time finding someone to go with me. T F

T F

44. During the past week, I felt hopeful about the future more than half the time.
45. Every time an election year rolls around, I learn anew that politicians cannot be trusted. T F
46. If I needed a place to stay for a week because of an emergency (for example, the electricity was

out in my apartment or house), I could easily   T   F
find someone who would put me up.

47. Whenever an elevator stops too long on a floor   T   F
above where I am waiting, I soon start to feel
irritated.   T   F

48. I have no one with whom I can share my most
private worries and fears.   T   F

49. When I'm around someone I don't like, I find it
hard not to be rude to him or her.

50. During the past week, there were three or more   T   F
days when I felt that my life has been a failure.

51. When I see a very overweight person walking   T   F
down the street, I wonder why such people are
so lacking in self-control.   T   F

52. If I was sick, there would be almost no one to
help me with daily chores.   T   F

53. When riding as a passenger in the front seat of
a car, I try to be alert for obstacles ahead.   T   F

54. There is someone I can turn to for advice about
handling problems with my family.   T   F

55. During the past week, I felt fearful more than   T   F
half the time.

56. When someone criticizes something I have   T   F
done, it makes me feel annoyed.

57. I am as good at doing things as most other
people are.   T   F

58. When involved in an argument, I can feel my
heart pounding and I breathe harder.   T   F

59. If I decided one afternoon that I would like to   T   F
go to a movie that evening, I could easily find
someone to go with me.   T   F

60. There were three or more nights during the past
week when my sleep was restless.

61. I have a lot of privacy at work.   T   F

62. When a friend or coworker disagrees with me, I
am apt to get into an argument with him or her.

63. When I need suggestions on how to deal with a personal problem, I know someone I can turn to.   T   F

64. When someone else is speaking very slowly during a conversation, I am apt to finish his or her sentences.   T   F

65. If I needed an emergency loan of one hundred dollars, there is someone (friend, relative, or acquaintance) I could get it from.   T   F
                                                                                                                           T   F

66. It's fear of being caught that keeps most people from sneaking into a movie theater without paying.   T   F

67. During the past week I was happy more than half the time.   T   F

68. Hearing news of another terrorist attack makes me feel like lashing out.   T   F

69. In general, people do not have much confidence in me.   T   F

70. When talking with my significant other, I often find my thoughts racing ahead to what I plan to say next.   T   F

71. Most people I know do not enjoy the same things I do.   T   F

72. At times in the past, when I was really angry, I threw things or slammed a door.   T   F

73. There is someone I could turn to for advice about making career plans or changing my job.   T   F

74. During the past week, there were three or more days when I talked less than usual.   T   F
                                                                                                                           T   F

75. At home or during leisure activities off the job, I have a lot of privacy.   T   F

76. The little annoyances of everyday life often seem to get under my skin.   T   F

77. I don't often get invited to do things with others.   T   F

78. When I disapprove of a friend's behavior, I usually let him or her know about it.   T   F

79. Most of my friends are more successful at making changes in their lives than I am.   T   F

80. During the past week, I felt lonely more than   T   F
    half the time.

81. I have very little control over how I spend my
    time at work.

82. When checking in at an airline ticket counter, I   T   F
    generally leave the seat assignment to the agent.

83. If I had to go out of town for a few weeks, it   T   F
    would be difficult to find someone who would
    look after my house or apartment (the plants,   T   F
    pets, garden, etc.).

84. I feel grouchy some of the time during nearly   T   F
    every day of the week.

85. There is really no one I can trust to give me   T   F
    good financial advice.

86. During the past week, there were three or more   T   F
    days when people were unfriendly.

87. If someone bumps into me in a store, I am apt
    to feel irritated at the person's clumsiness.   T   F

88. If I wanted to have lunch with someone, I could
    easily find a person to join me.   T   F

89. When my significant other is preparing a meal,
    I keep an eye on things to make sure nothing   T   F
    burns or cooks too long.

90. I am more satisfied with my life than most   T   F
    people are with theirs.

91. I enjoyed life more than half the time during the
    past week.

92. At home and during leisure activities, I don't   T   F
    have much control over how I spend my time.

93. If a friend calls at the last minute, pleading that   T   F
    he or she is "too tired to go out tonight," and I'm
    stuck with a pair of twenty-dollar tickets, I will   T   F
    tell my friend how inconsiderate he or she is.

94. If I were stranded ten miles from home, there is   T   F
    someone I could call who would come to get me.

95. When I recall something that angered me in the   T   F
    past, I feel angry all over again.

96. No one I know would throw a birthday party   T   F
    for me.

97. Many of the people I see walking around shop-   T   F
    ping malls are just wasting time.
98. It would be difficult to find someone who
    would lend me his or her car for a few hours.   T   F
99. During the past week, I had crying spells dur-
    ing three or more days.
100. When someone is hogging the conversation at   T   F
     a party, I make it a point to put him or her
     down.   T   F
101. If a family crisis arose, it would be difficult to
     find someone who could give me good advice   T   F
     about how to handle it.
102. When I have to work with incompetent people,   T   F
     it ticks me off to have to put up with them.
103. I am closer to my friends than most other   T   F
     people are to theirs.
104. During the past week, I felt sad more than half
     the time.   T   F
105. I have very little latitude in making decisions at
     work.   T   F
106. When my spouse (boyfriend/girlfriend) is going
     to get me a birthday present, I usually prefer to   T   F
     pick it out myself.
107. There is at least one person I know whose advice
     I really trust.   T   F
108. When I hold a poor opinion of someone, I will
     probably let him or her know about it.   T   F
109. If I needed some help in moving to a new house T   F
     or apartment, I would have a hard time finding
     someone to help me.   T   F
110. During the past week, there were three or more
     days when I felt that people disliked me.   T   F
111. In most arguments, I am the angrier one.
112. I have had a hard time keeping pace with my
     friends.

113. During the past week, I could not "get going" on three or more days.

114. At home or in my leisure activities, I have very little latitude in making decisions.

SOCIAL SUPPORT

The most direct indicator of the quality and quantity of your relationships is your score on the forty social support questions. Your total social support score is made up of four distinct kinds of support:

- *emotional support:* the degree to which you have someone who can help you deal with emotional problems
- *belonging support:* the degree to which you have a network of family and friends to do things with
- *tangible support:* the degree to which you have someone who can help you meet material needs (for example, a ride to the airport)
- *self-esteem:* the degree to which your relationships boost self-worth

To evaluate *emotional support,* give one point for each of these answers:

2-T	63-T
16-F	73-T
31-F	85-F
48-F	101-F
54-T	107-T

To measure *belonging support* from networks of family and friends, give one point for each of these answers:

13-T	59-T
21-T	71-F
29-F	77-F
34-T	88-T
43-F	96-F

To score *tangible support,* give one point for each of these answers:

5-T	65-T
25-F	83-F
41-F	94-T
46-T	98-F
52-F	109-F

To tally *self-esteem,* give one point for each of these answers:

7-F	69-F
11-T	79-F
23-T	90-T
36-F	103-T
57-T	112-F

Add up the components for your relationship scores:

Emotional Support	_____
Belonging Support	_____
Tangible Support	_____
Self-Esteem	_____
Total Social Support	_____

The higher your social support score, the better your relationships. If your total score is below 28 (out of a possible 40), it would be wise to seek strategies to improve your relationships. To do so would increase the likelihood of your becoming (or remaining) a highly healthy person. If any component of total social support is seven or less, that particular component needs the most immediate attention.

DEPRESSION

The loss of motivation and energy caused by depression can diminish, damage, or destroy relationships—and can reduce one's health. You cannot be highly healthy and be depressed; they cannot coexist. This questionnaire can help you evaluate any depression that might be in your soul. To score your level of *depression,* give yourself one point for each of these answers:

3-T	60-T
8-T	67-F
14-T	74-T
18-F	80-T
26-T	86-T
32-T	91-F
37-T	99-T
44-F	104-T
50-T	110-T
55-T	113-T

If your depression score is 5 or higher, your level of depression is a matter of concern and is very likely not only affecting your relationships but also reducing your chances of being a highly healthy person.

HOSTILITY

The questionnaire can help you screen for hostility as it comes to expression in cynicism, anger, and aggression. Each of these characteristics can lead you to mistrust—or be mistrusted by—others, thus damaging your relationships and your health.

To tabulate your level of *cynicism,* give yourself one point for each of these answers:

6-T	53-T
10-T	66-T
17-T	70-T
24-T	82-F
35-T	89-T
45-T	97-T
51-T	106-T

To record your level of *anger,* give yourself one point for each of these answers:

1-T	68-T
15-F	76-T
22-T	84-T
33-T	87-T
40-F	95-T
47-T	102-T
56-T	111-T
58-T	

To total your level of *aggression,* give yourself one point for each of these answers:

4-T	62-T
12-T	64-T
20-T	72-T
28-F	78-T
30-F	93-T
38-T	100-T
42-T	108-T
49-T	

Add up your total hostility score:

Cynicism	____
Anger	____
Aggression	____
Total Hostility	____

If your total hostility score is above sixteen, then your level of hostility is impairing your relationships—and that, I would predict, can keep you from becoming a highly healthy person.

STRESS

Finally, the questionnaire will help you screen for high levels of stress at home or at play. Once again, give yourself one point for each of these answers:

19-T   92-T
39-T   114-T
75-F

A score of three or more suggests that work or leisure stress is impairing your relationships.

At Pastor Randy Frazee's request, the reader may NOT photocopy the spiritual life profile found on these pages. This profile is intended for the reader's personal use only.

The most recent version of the Christian Life Profile (on which this spiritual life profile is based) can be obtained by contacting Pantego Bible Church, 8001 Anderson Blvd., Fort Worth, Texas 76120; by phone at 1-866-pantego [toll-free] or 817-274-1315; via e-mail at CLP@pantego.org; or on the Internet at www.pantego.org/mall/details.cfm?id=50.

THE SPIRITUAL WHEEL

Broad Category	Subcategory	20 Core Competencies
LOVE GOD	**(Beliefs & Practices)**	1. Personal God 2. Compassion 3. Stewardship 4. Worship 5. Prayer 6. Single-mindedness 7. Faith Community 8. Giving Away My Time 9. Giving Away My Money 10. Giving Away My Life
LOVE NEIGHBOR	**(Virtues)**	1. Love 2. Joy 3. Peace 4. Patience 5. Kindness/Goodness 6. Faithfulness 7. Gentleness 8. Self-control 9. Hope 10. Humility

PERSONAL ASSESSMENT

	Does not apply at all		Applies somewhat		Applies completely
1. I believe that God has a purpose for my life.	0	1	2	3	4	5
2. God calls me to be involved in the lives of the poor and suffering.	0	1	2	3	4	5
3. I believe that everything I am—or own—comes from God and belongs to God.	0	1	2	3	4	5
4. I thank God daily for who he is and for what he is doing in my life.	0	1	2	3	4	5
5. I seek God's will through prayer.	0	1	2	3	4	5
6. I desire God to be first in my life.	0	1	2	3	4	5
7. I have close relationships with others in my faith community who have influence in my life's direction.	0	1	2	3	4	5
8. I invest my time in others by praying for them.	0	1	2	3	4	5
9. I give away 10 percent or more of my income to God's work.	0	1	2	3	4	5
10. I am living out God's purposes for my life.	0	1	2	3	4	5
11. God's grace enables me to forgive people who have hurt me.	0	1	2	3	4	5
12. I have inner contentment even when things go wrong.	0	1	2	3	4	5
13. I know God forgives me.	0	1	2	3	4	5
14. I do not get angry with God when I have to endure suffering.	0	1	2	3	4	5
15. I would never keep money that didn't belong to me.	0	1	2	3	4	5
16. I take unpopular stands when my faith dictates.	0	1	2	3	4	5
17. I consider my own shortcomings when faced with the failures of others.	0	1	2	3	4	5
18. I am not addicted to any substances—whether food, caffeine, tobacco, alcohol, or chemical.	0	1	2	3	4	5

	Does not apply at all	Applies somewhat	Applies completely

19. I think a great deal about heaven and what God is preparing for me as a person of faith.
`0   1   2   3   4   5`

20. As a child of God, I do not think too highly or lowly of myself.
`0   1   2   3   4   5`

21. I believe that pain and suffering can often bring me closer to God.
`0   1   2   3   4   5`

22. I believe I am responsible before God to show compassion to the sick and imprisoned.
`0   1   2   3   4   5`

23. I believe that people of faith should live a sacrificial life, not be driven by pursuit of material things.
`0   1   2   3   4   5`

24. I attend religious services and worship with other believers each week.
`0   1   2   3   4   5`

25. I regularly admit to God the things I do wrong.
`0   1   2   3   4   5`

26. I see every aspect of my life and work as service to God.
`0   1   2   3   4   5`

27. I participate in a small faith group that really knows me and supports me.
`0   1   2   3   4   5`

28. I spend a good deal of time helping others who have physical, emotional, or other kinds of needs.
`0   1   2   3   4   5`

29. I regularly give money to serve and help others.
`0   1   2   3   4   5`

30. I give up what I want to meet the needs of others.
`0   1   2   3   4   5`

31. I rejoice when good things happen to other people.
`0   1   2   3   4   5`

32. Circumstances do not dictate my mood.
`0   1   2   3   4   5`

33. I am not angry with God, myself, or others.
`0   1   2   3   4   5`

34. I am known to maintain honesty and integrity when under pressure.
`0   1   2   3   4   5`

35. I am known as a person who speaks words of kindness to those in need of encouragement.
`0   1   2   3   4   5`

	Does not apply at all		Applies somewhat		Applies completely	
36. I discipline my thoughts based on my faith.	0	1	2	3	4	5
37. I am known as a person who is sensitive to the needs of others.	0	1	2	3	4	5
38. I do not burst out toward others in anger.	0	1	2	3	4	5
39. I am confident that God is working everything out for my good regardless of the circumstances today.	0	1	2	3	4	5
40. I am not known as a person who brags.	0	1	2	3	4	5
41. I believe that God is actively involved in my life.	0	1	2	3	4	5
42. I believe that I should stand up for those who cannot stand up for themselves.	0	1	2	3	4	5
43. I believe that I should give at least 10 percent of my income to God's work.	0	1	2	3	4	5
44. I give God credit for all that I am and all that I possess.	0	1	2	3	4	5
45. Prayer is a central part of my daily life.	0	1	2	3	4	5
46. I spend time each day reading God's Word and praying.	0	1	2	3	4	5
47. I allow others in my faith community to hold me accountable for my actions.	0	1	2	3	4	5
48. I give away my time to serve and help others in my community.	0	1	2	3	4	5
49. My first priority in spending is to support God's work.	0	1	2	3	4	5
50. I give away things I possess, when I am so led by God.	0	1	2	3	4	5
51. I demonstrate love equally toward people of all races.	0	1	2	3	4	5
52. I am excited about the sense of purpose I have for my life.	0	1	2	3	4	5
53. I forgive people who deeply hurt me.	0	1	2	3	4	5

	Does not apply at all		Applies somewhat		Applies completely

54. I always put matters into God's hands when I am under pressure. 0 1 2 3 4 5

55. I give to others, expecting nothing in return. 0 1 2 3 4 5

56. I follow God even when it involves suffering. 0 1 2 3 4 5

57. I am known for not raising my voice. 0 1 2 3 4 5

58. I do not have sexual relationships that are contrary to the teaching of my faith community. 0 1 2 3 4 5

59. My hope in God increases through my daily pursuit to follow his teachings. 0 1 2 3 4 5

60. I am willing to make any of my faults known to people in my faith community who care for me. 0 1 2 3 4 5

61. I believe God enables me to do things I could not or would not otherwise do. 0 1 2 3 4 5

62. I believe that I should not purchase everything I can afford, in order that at least some of my discretionary money can be available to help those in need. 0 1 2 3 4 5

63. I believe God will bless people of faith now and in the life to come for their good deeds. 0 1 2 3 4 5

64. I am not ashamed for others to know that I worship God. 0 1 2 3 4 5

65. I seek to grow closer to God by listening to him either in prayer or by reading his Word. 0 1 2 3 4 5

66. I value a simple lifestyle over one cluttered with activities and material possessions. 0 1 2 3 4 5

67. I daily pray for and support other people of my faith community. 0 1 2 3 4 5

68. I regularly volunteer in my community. 0 1 2 3 4 5

69. My spending habits do not keep me from giving what I feel I should give to God. 0 1 2 3 4 5

70. I serve God through my daily work. 0 1 2 3 4 5

71. I frequently give up what I want for the sake of others. 0 1 2 3 4 5

	Does not apply at all		Applies somewhat		Applies completely	
72. I can be content with the money and possessions I now have.	0	1	2	3	4	5
73. I have an inner peace from God.	0	1	2	3	4	5
74. I keep my composure even when people or circumstances irritate me.	0	1	2	3	4	5
75. I help others who are in trouble or who cannot help themselves.	0	1	2	3	4	5
76. I follow through on commitments I have made to God.	0	1	2	3	4	5
77. I allow people to make mistakes.	0	1	2	3	4	5
78. I control my tongue.	0	1	2	3	4	5
79. My hope for the future is not found in my health or wealth—because both are so uncertain—but in God.	0	1	2	3	4	5
80. I am not upset when my achievements are not recognized.	0	1	2	3	4	5

SCORING TABLE FOR THE SPIRITUAL LIFE PROFILE

Go back through your personal assessment; take your score for each question and transfer it to this table. For example, if you answered question #1 (I believe that God has a purpose for my life) by saying that this statement "applies somewhat" (a score of 3), then place the score of 3 by number 1 below. Repeat this process for each question on the personal assessment. When you have placed your scores in each of the blanks, add the scores for each line and place this sum on the 0–20 point scale of that line. When you are done, add your score for each section and place it in the box below each section.

A Discipleship Tool to Assess Christian Beliefs, Practices, and Virtues

1. ___	21. ___	41. ___	61. ___	Personal God	0....5....10....15....20
2. ___	22. ___	42. ___	62. ___	Compassion	0....5....10....15....20
3. ___	23. ___	43. ___	63. ___	Stewardship	0....5....10....15....20
4. ___	24. ___	44. ___	64. ___	Worship	0....5....10....15....20
5. ___	25. ___	45. ___	65. ___	Prayer	0....5....10....15....20
6. ___	26. ___	46. ___	66. ___	Single-mindedness	0....5....10....15....20
7. ___	27. ___	47. ___	67. ___	Faith Community	0....5....10....15....20
8. ___	28. ___	48. ___	68. ___	Giving Away My Time	0....5....10....15....20
9. ___	29. ___	49. ___	69. ___	Giving Away My Money	0....5....10....15....20
10. ___	30. ___	50. ___	70. ___	Giving Away My Life	0....5....10....15....20

Total Score in Beliefs and Practices [ ] 0...40...80...120...160...200

11. ___	31. ___	51. ___	71. ___	Love	0....5....10....15....20
12. ___	32. ___	52. ___	72. ___	Joy	0....5....10....15....20
13. ___	33. ___	53. ___	73. ___	Peace	0....5....10....15....20
14. ___	34. ___	54. ___	74. ___	Patience	0....5....10....15....20
15. ___	35. ___	55. ___	75. ___	Kindness/Goodness	0....5....10....15....20
16. ___	36. ___	56. ___	76. ___	Faithfulness	0....5....10....15....20
17. ___	37. ___	57. ___	77. ___	Gentleness	0....5....10....15....20
18. ___	38. ___	58. ___	78. ___	Self-control	0....5....10....15....20
19. ___	39. ___	59. ___	79. ___	Hope	0....5....10....15....20
20. ___	40. ___	60. ___	80. ___	Humility	0....5....10....15....20

Total Score in Virtues [ ] 0...40...80...120...160...200

NOTES

Chapter One: What Is a Highly Healthy Person?

24: *"Value this time"*: From *City Slickers,* Columbia Pictures, 1991; screenplay by Lowell Ganz and Babaloo Mandel.

25: *"One such patient"*: Terrie is not her real name. Throughout this book the name, age, and sometimes even the gender of my patients have been changed to protect their confidentiality. In fact, when I was in practice, I would not reveal to anyone outside the practice that I was someone's doctor. I treasure the doctor-patient relationship and would not abuse it—especially for a document as public as this book!

28: *"I think that true health"*: Reported by D. Dean Patton, M.D., personal communication, 10 January 2001.

29: *"human wholeness or health"*: John Wilkinson, *The Bible and Healing: A Medical and Theological Commentary* (Grand Rapids: Eerdmans, 2002), 7.

29: *"The LORD gives strength"*: Psalm 29:11.

29: *"A cheerful heart"*: Proverbs 17:22.

30: *"When I kept silent"*: Psalm 32:3–4.

30: *"Dear friend"*: 3 John 2.

30: *"Sermon on the Mount"*: Matthew 5:3–12; see also Luke 6:20–26.

Chapter Two: Testing Your Four Wheels of Health

33: *"The essence of true health"*: Michael Freeney, personal communication, 6 January 2001.

38: *"infused with purpose, contentment, and joy"*: See John 10:10.

43: *"Researchers have shown that the brain"*: Reported on the Web at www.sfn.org/content/Publications/BrainBriefings/exercise.html.

43: *"Those who take the time to teach others"*: L. F. Zhang, "Approaches and thinking styles in teaching," *Journal of Psychology* (September 2001): 135(5):547–61; J. Merrell, "You don't do it for nothing: Women's experiences of volunteering in two community well woman clinics," *Journal of Health and Social Care in the Community* (January 2000): 8(1):31–39; J. Hainsworth and J. Barlow, "Volunteers' experiences of becoming arthritis self-management lay leaders: 'It's almost as if I've stopped aging and started to get younger!'" *Arthritis and Rheumatism* (August 2001): 45(4):378–83.

Chapter Three: Set a Wise Balance in Your Life

56: *"the most overworked nation"*: Silja J.A. Talvi, "Lights out for long hours?" *The Christian Science Monitor* (17 December 2001); on the Web at www.csmonitor.com/2001/1217/p15s1-wmwo.html.

57: *"excessive work hours are not safe"*: See the article on the Web at www.ama-assn.org/ama/pub/article/1616-5665.html.

57: *"effects of sleep loss"*: See the report on the Web at http://news.bbc.co.uk/hi/english/health/newsid_930000/930615.stm.

57: *"men who slept five hours"*: See Y. Liu and H. Tanaka, "Overtime work, insufficient sleep, and risk of non-fatal acute myocardial infarction in Japanese men," *Occupational and Environmental Medicine* (2002): 59:447–51.

57: *"The phenomenon was first identified"*: See the report on the Web at www.ilocis.org/sample1.html.

57: *Tanzi*: Rudolph E. Tanzi and Ann B. Parson, *Decoding Darkness: The Search for the Genetic Causes of Alzheimer's Disease* (Cambridge, Mass.: Perseus, 2000).

57: *"brain must be exercised"*: R. P. Friedland et al., "Patients with Alzheimer's disease have reduced activities in midlife compared with healthy control-group members," *Proceedings of the National Academy of Sciences of the United States of America* (2001): 98:3440–45.

57: *"A 2002 study"*: R. S. Wilson et al., "Participation in cognitively stimulating activities and risk of incident Alzheimer disease," *Journal of the American Medical Association* (2002): 287(6):742–48.

Chapter Four: Be Proactive in Preventing Disease

64: *"They're not 'wallowers'"*: See the article on the Web at www.savannahnow.com/features/aging/part2/livingto100.shtml.

65–66: *"group of more than one hundred centenarians"*: These findings are reported on The New England Centenarian Study Website. See the report on the Web at http://www.bumc.bu.edu/Departments/HomeMain.aasp?DepartmentID=361.

66: *Perls*: Thomas Perls and Margery Hutter Silver, with John Lauerman, *Living to 100: Lessons in Living to Your Maximum Potential at Any Age* (New York: Basic Books, 2000).

67–68: *"leading causes of death in the United States"*: See the report of The Centers for Disease Control and Prevention at www.cdc.gov/nchs/fastats/lcod.htm.

68: *"died from breast cancer"*: See the report of The Centers for Disease Control and Prevention at www.cdc.gov/nchs/fastats/women.htm.

69: *"alleged ill effects"*: Elizabeth M. Whelan, "Inverted priorities: Health hazards in women's magazines," *Priorities for Health* (1992), vol. 4, no. 4; on the Web at www.acsh.org/publications/priorities/0404/hazards.html.

70: *"Tobacco companies"*: Marilyn Gardner, "Cigarette companies blow smoke in women's eyes," *The Christian Science Monitor* (8 January 1998); on the Web at www.csmonitor.com/durable/1998/01/08/feat/feat.1.html.

70: *"I have been an accomplice"*: Joe Eszterhas, writing in *The New York Times* (9 August 2002, op-ed page).

70: *"Don't you know"*: 1 Corinthians 3:16–18.

71: *"from my Website"*: Turn your Internet browser to www.highlyhealthy.net. Click on this chapter, and then locate and click on this hyperlink.

72: *"at my Website"*: Turn your Internet browser to www.highlyhealthy.net. Click on this chapter, and then locate and click on this hyperlink.

73: *"Health care costs"*: Reported in D. Allison et al., "Annual Deaths Attributable to Obesity in the United States," *Journal of the American Medical Association* (1999): 282(16):1530-38.

75: *"To maintain cardiovascular"*: National Academy of Sciences, *Dietary Reference Intakes for Energy, Carbohydrate, Fiber, Fat, Fatty Acids, Cholesterol, Protein, and Amino Acids* (Washington, D.C.: The National Academies Press, 2002).

75: *"Your fitness level"*: J. Myers et al., "Exercise capacity and mortality among men referred for exercise testing," *New England Journal of Medicine* (2002): 346(11): 793–801.

77: *"Married people are"*: Facts and Stats: Benefits of Marriage, Friends First (2002); on the Web at www.friendsfirst.org/factmarriage.html.

77: *"That's the finding"*: Dr. Robert H. Coombs, professor of biobehavioral sciences at the University of California at Los Angeles (UCLA), conducted a review of more than 130 published empirical studies measuring how marital status affects personal well-being. Reported in Glenn T. Stanton, "What's Marriage Got to Do With It?"; on the Web at www.family.org/cforum/research/papers/a0002965.html.

77: *"condoms were proven"*: National Institutes of Health study panel; on the Web at reproline.jhu.edu/english/6read/6issues/6network/v21-2/nt2126.htm.

78: *"high school seniors were virgins"*: The Centers for Disease Control, "Trends in sexual risk behaviors among high school students—United States, 1991 –2001," *Morbidity and Mortality Weekly Report* (27 September 2002); 51(38):856–59.

80: *"Americans are confused"*: Cited in Alicia M. Lukachko, "Consumers Unaware of Leading Causes of Premature Death" (17 April 2000), American Council on Science and Health editorial (www.acsh.org).

80: *"Cigarette smoking also"*: Lukachko, "Consumers Unaware of Leading Causes of Premature Death."

81: *"alternative therapy"*: I've written extensively about this topic in *Alternative Medicine: The Christian Handbook* (Grand Rapids: Zondervan, 2001). In this book, Dónal O'Mathúna, Ph.D., and I discuss the evidence supporting the thirty-six most common alternative therapies used in America (everything from acupuncture to yoga) and fifty-six common herbs, vitamins, and supplements (everything from aloe to zinc).

81: *"Some alternative therapies are contraindicated"*: One of the most accurate and complete sources of information on natural medicines (herbs, vitamins, and supplements) is the *Natural Medicines Comprehensive Database* (Therapeutic Research Faculty, 1999). The book can be ordered from most bookstores or accessed via the Internet at www.naturaldatabase.com. This is a subscription Website—but well worth the cost. You may want to check your   public library to see if they have a copy. Another subscription Website—www.ConsumerLab.com—gives independent lab results on a number of commonly used herbs, vitamins, and supplements. This site lists the ones that have passed a number of quality tests. The annual subscription is less than the cost of a single bottle of most herbal preparations.

81: *"Even more surprising"*: Reported in Consumers Union, "The mainstreaming of alternative medicine," *Consumer Reports* (May 2000): 17–25.

82: *"Seat belts are a priority"*: Buckle Up America; can be viewed on the Web at www.buckleupamerica.org/; quotes can be found at www.nhtsa.dot.gov/people/injury/airbags/buckleplan/buckleup/keymess.html.

85: *"go to my Website"*: Turn your Internet browser to www.highlyhealthy.net. Click on this chapter, and then locate and click on this hyperlink.

85: *"find this profile"*: Turn your Internet browser to www.highlyhealthy.net. Click on this chapter, and then locate and click on this hyperlink.

86: *"via my Website"*: Turn your Internet browser to www.highlyhealthy.net. Click on this chapter, and then locate and click on this hyperlink.

88: *Harvard Center for Cancer Prevention*: The Harvard Center for Cancer Prevention is a research and education center based at Harvard School of Public Health. This center promotes prevention as the primary approach to cancer control. Its cancer-risk calculators are based on the findings of the Risk Index Working Group at Harvard University.

89: *"find this site"*: Turn your Internet browser to www.highlyhealthy.net. Click on this chapter, and then locate and click on this hyperlink.

Chapter Five: Practice Acceptance and Letting Go

93: *"Researchers in San Diego"*: Reported in J. McCauley et al., "Clinical characteristics of women with a history of child abuse: Unhealed wounds," *Journal of the American Medical Association* (1997): 277(17):1362–68.

101: *Virgina Williams*: Redford Williams and Virginia Williams, *Anger Kills: 17 Strategies for Controlling the Hostility That Can Harm Your Health* (New York: HarperCollins, 1998).

101: *"In your anger"*: Ephesians 4:26.

102: *"If we claim"*: 1 John 1:8–10.

103: *"He who covers"*: Proverbs 17:9.

104: *"If you are offering"*: Matthew 5:23–24.

105: *"People who forgive themselves"*: See L. L. Toussaint et al., "Forgiveness and health: Age differences in a U.S. probability sample," *Journal of Adult Development* (October 2001): 8(4):249–57.

106: *"Father, forgive them"*: Luke 23:34.

107–8: *"Dear friends, do not"*: 1 Peter 4:12–13.

109: *"We also rejoice"*: Romans 5:3–5.

108: *"So then, just as you"*: Colossians 2:6–7.

108: *"Let your gentleness"*: Philippians 4:4–7.

109: *"comforts us in all"*: 2 Corinthians 1:4.

Chapter Six: Lighten Your Load

111: *"Rand researchers"*: Reported in M. A. Schuster et al., "A national survey of stress reactions after the September 11, 2001, terrorist attacks," *New England Journal of Medicine* (15 November 2001): 345(20):1507–1512.

112: *"researchers from Johns Hopkins"*: Reported in L. R. Yanek, T. F. Moy, and L. C. Becker, Abstract #103966: "General well-being is strongly protective against future coronary heart disease events in an apparently healthy high-risk population," Johns Hopkins Office of Communications and Public Affairs (12 November 2001); can be viewed on the Web at www.hopkinsmedicine.org/press/2001/november/011112.htm.

112: *"a patient's expectations"*: M. V. Mondloch, D. C. Cole, and J. W. Frank, "Does how you do depend on how you think you'll do? A systematic review of the evidence for a relation between patients' recovery expectations and health outcomes," *Canadian Medical Association Journal* (24 July 2001): 165(2):174–79.

113: *"constantly being tested"*: See Job 23:10 and 1 Peter 1:7, for example.

114: *"can be accessed via"*: Turn your Internet browser to www.highlyhealthy.net. Click on this chapter, and then locate and click on this hyperlink.

114–15: *"researchers at Duke University"*: Reported in J. A. Blumenthal et al., "Usefulness of psychosocial treatment of mental stress-induced myocardial ischemia in men," *The American Journal of Cardiology* (15 January 2002): 89(2):164–68.

118: *"at my Website"*: Turn your Internet browser to www.highlyhealthy.net. Click on this chapter, and then locate and click on this hyperlink.

120: *"Our findings suggest"*: J. A. Blumenthal et al., "Effects of exercise training on older patients with major depression," *Archives of Internal Medicine* (25 October 1999): 159(19):2349–56.

120: *"Dr. Blumenthal speculated"*: Reported in J. A. Blumenthal et al., "Depression and vascular function in older adults. Evaluating the benefits of exercise in a new study at Duke University," *North Carolina Medical Journal* (March–April 2001): 62(2):95–98.

120: *"going to my Website"*: Turn your Internet browser to www.highlyhealthy.net. Click on this chapter, and then locate and click on this hyperlink.

122: *"You can access"*: Turn your Internet browser to www.highlyhealthy.net. Click on this chapter, and then locate and click on this hyperlink.

122: *"Among their findings"*: Thomas Perls and Margery Hutter Silver, with John Lauerman, *Living to 100: Lessons in Living to Your Maximum Potential at Any Age* (New York: Basic Books, 2000).

122: *"nuns who had articulated"*: Reported by Edward M. Eveld, "Nun Such: Sisters Have Much to Teach about Living Long, Happy Lives," *The Gazette*—Colorado Springs (30 June 2001).

122: *"Hope really pays"*: Reported in "Nun Such."

123: *"I think personality"*: Reported in "Nun Such."

123:    *"A man can do"*: Ecclesiastes 2:24–26.

123:    *"There is a God-shaped"*: Quoted at www.billbright.com/intellectual/purpose.html.

123:    *"Hope is the companion"*: Quoted at The Quotations Page; on the Web at www.quotationspage.com.

126:    *"Writer G. K. Chesterton"*: Frederic and Mary Ann Brussat, "Countdown to Thanksgiving: 26 Ways to Practice Giving Thanks," *Spirituality and Health;* on the Web at www.spiritualityhealth.com/newsh/items/article/item_2914.html.

126:    *Breathnach*: Sarah Ban Breathnach, *Simple Abundance: A Daybook of Comfort and Joy* (New York: Warner, 1995).

126:    *"first-ever conference"*: For more information, visit www.templeton.org/humbleapproach/Gratitude/default.asp.

126–27:   *"kept gratitude lists"*: Reported in R. A. Emmons and C. A. Crumpler, "Gratitude as a human strength: Appraising the evidence," *Journal of Social and Clinical Psychology* (2000): 19(1)56–59.

127:    *"the grateful disposition"*: The studies are reviewed in: M. E. McCullough, R. A. Emmons, and J. A. Tsang, "The grateful disposition: A conceptual and empirical topography," *Journal of Personality and Social Psychology* (January 2002): 82(1):112–27.

127:    *"triggered positive feelings"*: Reported in B. L. Fredrickson and R. W. Levenson, "Positive emotions speed recovery from the cardiovascular sequelae of negative emotions," *Cognition & Emotion* (March 1998): 12(2):191–220.

127:    *"It may be easier"*: Quoted in Ann Japenga, "Can You Cope Better? Absolutely. And the secret may be as simple as learning to give thanks"; on the Web at http://webmd.lycos.com/content/article/1674.50615.

129:    *"ability to laugh"*: Reported in A. Clark, A. Seidler, and M. Miller, "Inverse association between sense of humor and coronary heart disease," *International Journal of Cardiology* (August 2001): 80(1):87–88.

129:    *"Laughter is no substitute"*: Quoted in Teri Walsh, "Funny Heart Protection," *Prevention Magazine* online; on the Web at www.prevention.com/cda/column/0,1210,1098,00.html.

129:    *"Researchers at Marywood University"*: Reported in Victor Parachin, "Ten Stress Busters That Really Work"; can be viewed on the Web at www.finalthoughts.com/rc_html/main/article.asp?ID=109&Resource=4.

131:    *"That sensation"*: Quoted in Mark Moran, "Kindness Is Contagious"; on the Web at http://my.webmd.com/content/article/3606.609.

131:    *Bennett*: William J. Bennett, *The Book of Virtues: A Treasury of Great Moral Stories* (New York: Simon & Schuster, 1993).

131:    *"The study of elevation"*: Moran, "Kindness Is Contagious."

131:    *"school-based education program"*: Teachers or parents interested in the "Kindness Is Contagious" program can purchase a two-volume guidebook for $20. Write to Stop Violence Coalition, 301 East Armour, Suite 440, Kansas City, Missouri 64111.

132:    *"The feedback we got"*: Quoted in Moran, "Kindness Is Contagious."

Chapter Seven: Avoid Loneliness

137: *"It is not good"*: Genesis 2:7, 18.

139: *"Community is in short supply"*: Bishop Edmond Lee Browning, *A Year of Days with the Book of Common Prayer* (New York: Ballantine, 1997), January 22.

139: *"Overall, the research"*: Reported in Barna Updates, "Most People Seek Control, Adventure and Peace in Their Lives" (1 August 2000); on the Web at http://www.barna.org/cgibin/PagePressRelease.asp?PressReleaseID=68& Reference=B.

140: *"The researchers concluded"*: Reported in M. G. Marmot et al., "Epidemiologic studies of coronary heart disease and stroke in Japanese men living in Japan, Hawaii, and California: Prevalence of coronary and hypertensive heart disease and associated risk factors," *American Journal of Epidemiology* (1975): 102(6):514–25.

140: *"these risks were additive"*: Reported in T. E. Oxman, D. H. Fremman, and E. D. Manheimer, "Lack of social participation or religious strength and comfort as risk factors for death after cardiac surgery in the elderly," *Psychosomatic Medicine* (1995): 57:5–15.

140: *"Swedish researchers"*: Reported by Kristina Orth-Gomer, M.D., of the Karolinska Institute in Sweden, quoted in Dean Ornish, *Love and Survival* (New York: HarperPerennial, 1998), 186–87.

143: *"the perception of love"*: Reported in L. G. Russek and G. E. Schwartz, "Perceptions of parental caring predict health status in midlife: A 35-year followup of the Harvard Mastery of Stress Study," *Psychosomatic Medicine* (1997): 59(2):144–49.

143: *"likely to end up with cancer"*: Reported in C. B. Thomas and K. R. Duszynski, "Closeness to parents and the family constellation in a prospective study of five disease states: Suicide, mental illness, malignant tumor, hypertension, and coronary heart disease," *John Hopkins Medical Journal* (1974): 134:251.

145: *"The wife's love"*: Reported in J. H. Medalie and U. Goldbourt, "Angina pectoris among 10,000 men. II. Psychological and other risk factors as evidenced by a multivariate analysis of a five-year incidence study," *American Journal of Medicine* (1976): 60(6):910–21.

145–46: *"three times as many ulcers"*: Reported in J. H. Medalie et al., "The importance of biopsychosocial factors in the development of duodenal ulcer in a cohort of middle-aged men," *American Journal of Epidemiology* (1992): 136(10):1280–87.

146: *"percentage of cancer survivors"*: Reported in J. Goodwin et al., "The effect of marital status on stage, treatment, and survival of cancer patients," *Journal of the American Medical Association* (1987): 258(21):3130–52.

146: *"Another study showed"*: Reported in R. Williams et al., "Prognostic importance of social and economic resources among medically treated patient with angiographically documented coronary artery disease," *Journal of the American Medical Association* (1992): 267(4):520–24.

146:   *"Perhaps a strong"*: A. Oswald and J. Gardner, "Is It Money or Marriage That Keeps People Alive?"; can be viewed on the Web at www.warwick.ac.uk/fac/soc/Economics/oswald/.

146:   *"those who constantly argued"*: Reported in J. K. Kiecolt-Glaser et al., "Marital conflict in older adults: endocrinological and immunological correlates," *Psychosomatic Medicine* (1997): 59:339–49.

146:   *"A study of newlyweds"*: Reported in J. Kiecolt-Glaser, R. Glaser, J. Cacioppo, and W. Malarkey, "Marital stress: Immunologic, neuroendocrine, and autonomic correlates," *Annals of the New York Academy of Sciences* (1998): 840:656–63; on the Web at http://pni.psychiatry. ohio-state.edu/jkg/newlywed.htm.

146:   *"who avoided divorce"*: Reported in L. J. Waite et al., "Does Divorce Make People Happy? Findings from a Study of Unhappy Marriages," (2002); on the Web at www.americanvalues.org/html/r-unhappy_ii.html.

147:   *"how integrated you are"*: Cited in Dean Ornish, *Love and Survival* (New York: HarperPerennial, 1998), 186–87.

148:   *"well connected to"*: Reported in Lester Berkman and Lisa Breslow, *Health and Ways of Living: The Alameda County Study* (New York: Oxford Univ. Press, 1983).

148:   *"Cardiologists at Columbia"*: Reported in R. B. Case et al., "Living alone after myocardial infarction. Impact on prognosis," *Journal of the American Medical Association* (1992): 267(4):515–19.

148:   *"were socially connected"*: Reported in R. B. Williams et al., "Prognostic importance of social and economic resources among medically treated patients with angiographically documented coronary artery disease," *Journal of the American Medical Association* (1992): 267(4):520–24.

148:   *"social support increases"*: Reported in S. Cohen et al., "Social ties and susceptibility to the common cold," *Journal of the American Medical Association* (1997): 277(24):1940–44.

149:   *"reduced religious attendance"*: Reported in G. R. Lee and M. Ishii-Kuntz, "Social interaction, loneliness, and emotional well-being among the elderly," *Research on Aging* (1987): 9:359–482.

149:   *"The research reviewed"*: Harold G. Koenig, Michael E. McCullough, and David B. Larson, *Handbook of Religion and Health* (New York: Oxford Univ. Press, 2000).

149:   *"Let us not give up"*: Hebrews 10:25.

150:   *"those who owned dogs"*: Reported in E. Friedmann and S. A. Thomas, "Pet ownership, social support, and one-year survival after acute myocardial infarction in the Cardiac Arrhythmia Suppression Trial (CAST)," *American Journal of Cardiology* (1995): 76:1213–17.

151:   *"6 percent of pet owners"*: Reported in E. Friedmann et al., "Animal companions and one-year survival of patients after discharge from a coronary care unit," *Public Health Reports* (1980): 95:307–12.

151:   *"Medicaid recipients"*: Reported in J. M. Siegel, "Stressful life events and use of physician services among the elderly: The moderating role of pet owner-ship," *Journal of Personality and Social Psychology* (1990): 58:1081–86.

152: *"one support person"*: Reported in N. Frasure-Smith and R. Prince, "Long-term follow-up of the Ischemic Heart Disease Life Stress Monitoring Program," *Psychosomatic Medicine* (1989): 51(5):485–513.

152: *"support group patients"*: Reported in D. Spiegel et al., "Effect of psychoso-cial treatment on survival of patient with metastatic breast cancer," *The Lancet* (1989): 2(8677):888–91.

152: *"Over the six years"*: Reported in F. I. Fawzy et al., "Malignant melanoma: Effects of an early structured psychiatric intervention, coping, and affective state on recurrence and survival six years later," *Archives of General Psychi-atry* (1993): 50:681–89.

152: *"instead thinking about"*: Reported in an interview with James J. Lynch, Ph.D., in Dean Ornish, *Love and Survival* (New York: Harper Perennial, 1998), 249–53.

152: *"the more love and support"*: Reported in C. E. Depner and B. Ingersoll-Dayton, "Supportive relationships in later life," *Psychology and Aging* (1988): 3(4):348–57.

154: *Williamses*: The Relationships Questionnaire is taken from Virginia Williams and Redford Williams, *Lifeskills* (New York: Random House, 1998).

Chapter Eight: Cultivate a True Spirituality

159: *"What does it take"*: Bishop Edmond Lee Browning, *A Year of Days with the Book of Common Prayer* (New York: Ballantine, 1997), January 24.

161: *"true spirituality"*: For more on true spirituality, see M. Crowther, M. Parker, W. Achenbaum, W. Larimore, and H. Koenig, "Rowe and Kahn's model of successful aging revisited: Positive spirituality—the forgotten fac-tor," *The Gerontologist* (2002): 42:613–20.

161: *"fruit of love"*: See Galatians 5:22–23.

161: *"Researchers have shown"*: Reported in M. M. Poloma and B. F. Pendleton, "The effects of prayer and prayer experiences on measures of general well-being," *Journal of Psychology and Theology* (1991): 19:71–83.

161: *"Persons with this"*: G. W. Allport and J. M. Ross, "Personal religious ori-entation and prejudice," *Journal of Personality and Social Psychology* (1967): 5:432–43.

161: *"ask not what they"*: Dale Matthews, with Connie Clark, *The Faith Factor: Proof of the Healing Power of Prayer* (New York: Viking, 1998), 54.

161: *"a major depression"*: Reported in H.G. Koenig, L. K. George, and B. L. Peterson, "Religiosity and remission of depression in medically ill older patients," *American Journal of Psychiatry* (1998): 155(4):536–42.

162: *"although they are slightly"*: Reported in Barna Updates, "People's Faith Fla-vor Influences How They See Themselves" (26 August 2002); on the Web at http://www.barna.org/cgi-bin/PagePressRelease.asp?PressReleaseID=119&Reference=B.

162: *"study of elderly patients"*: Reported in T. E. Oxman, D. H. Freeman, and E. D. Manheimer, "Lack of social participation or religious strength or comfort as risk factors for death after cardiac surgery in the elderly," *Psychosomatic Medicine* (1995): 57:5–15.

163: *"influential study variable"*: Reported in D. M. Zuckerman, S. V. Kasl, and A. M. Ostfeld, "Psychosocial predictors of mortality among the elderly poor," *American Journal of Epidemiology* (1984): 119:410–23.

164: *Benson*: Herbert Benson, with Miriam Z. Klipper, *The Relaxation Response* (New York: WholeCare, 2000).

164: *"national adult study"*: Reported in C. G. Ellison, "Religious involvement and subjective well-being," *Journal of Health and Social Behavior* (1991): 32:80–99.

164: *"levels of life satisfaction"*: Reported in C. G. Ellison, D. A. Gay, and T. A. Glass, "Does religious commitment contribute to individual life satisfaction?" *Social Forces* (1989): 68:100–123.

165: *Handbook of Religion*: Harold G. Koenig, Michael E. McCullough, and David B. Larson, *Handbook of Religion and Health* (New York: Oxford Univ. Press, 2000).

165: *"who attended religious services"*: Reported in R. Hummer, R. Rogers, C. Nam, and C. G. Ellison, "Religious involvement and U.S. adult mortality," *Demography* (1999): 36(2):273–85.

165: *"Duke researchers"*: Reported in D. B. Larson et al., "The impact of religion on man's blood pressure," *Journal of Religion and Health* (1989): 28(4):265–78.

165: *"Dartmouth researchers"*: Reported in Oxman, Freeman, and Manheimer, "Lack of social participation," *Psychosomatic Medicine* (1995): 57:5–15.

165: *"Duke researchers"*: Reported in H. G. Koenig and D. B. Larson, "Use of hospital services, religious attendance, and religious affiliation," *Southern Medical Journal* (1998): 91(10):925–32.

165: *"Duke University study"*: Reported in H. G. Koenig et al., "Modeling the cross-sectional relationships between religion, physical health, social support, and depressive symptoms," *American Journal of Geriatric Psychiatry* (1997): 5:131–43.

165–66: *"Levin's 1994 research"*: Reported in J. S. Levin, R. J. Taylor, and L. M. Chatters, "Differences in religiosity among older adults: Findings from four national surveys," *Journal of Gerontology: Social Sciences* (1994): 49:S137–S145.

166: *"Persons with high religious"*: Koenig et al., *Handbook*, 99.

167: *"only three schools"*: Reported in Jeff Sheler, "Drugs, Scalpel . . . and Faith?" *U.S. News & World Report* (2 July 2001), 46.

167–68: *"intercessory prayer can aid"*: Reported in Cullen Murphy, "Innocent Bystander; Physician Herbert Benson's Research on Benefits of Intercessory Prayer," *The Atlantic Monthly* (1 April 2001), 18.

168: *"who attended weekly services"*: Reported in Lan N. Nguyen, "Can Faith Help to Heal?" *The Seattle Times* (13 November 2001), E1.

168: *"A recent article"*: Reported in Kawanza L. Griffin, "Body and Soul; Some Doctors Adding Prayer to Treatment Equation," *Milwaukee Journal Sentinel* (5 November 2001), G1.

168: *"religious beliefs"*: Reported in Mary Rourke, "Is There a Place for Spirituality in Medicine?" *Los Angeles Times* (28 January 1997), E1.

168: *"On CBS"*: Reported by Julie Chen, *The Early Show* on the CBS Network (1 November 2001).

171: *Randy Frazee*: The most recent version of the CLP can be obtained by contacting Pantego Bible Church, 8001 Anderson Blvd., Fort Worth, Texas 76120; phone 1-866-pantego [toll-free] or 817-274-1315; via e-mail at CLP@pantego.org; or on the Internet at www.pantego.org/mall/details.cfm?id=50. Readers are reminded that this copyrighted material as presented in appendix 2 of this book is not to be photocopied.

Chapter Nine: See Yourself as Your Creator Sees You

176: *"We believe there are"*: Frank Minirth and Paul Meier, *Happiness Is a Choice: The Symptoms, Causes, and Cures of Depression* (Grand Rapids: Baker, 1994), 51.

177: *"most important one"*: Mark 12:28–31. Note that the Spiritual Life Profile (see page 272) is based on this precept.

178–79: *"you have searched me"*: Psalm 139:1–18.

179: *Minirth*: Frank Minirth, Paul Meier, Richard Meier, and Don Hawkins, *The Healthy Christian Life* (Grand Rapids: Baker, 1988), 102–3.

183: *"fairly strong relationship"*: Reported in L. Gruner, "The correlation of private, religious devotion practices and marital adjustment," *Journal of Comparative Family Studies* (1985): 16:47–59.

183: *"daily Bible reading"*: Reported in H. Ayele et al., "Religious activity improves life satisfaction for some physicians and older patients," *Journal of the American Geriatrics Society* (April 1999): 47(4):453–55.

183: *"hopefulness"*: Reported in E. Benzein, A. Norberg, and B. I. Saveman, "Hope: future imagined reality. The meaning of hope as described by a group of healthy Pentecostalists," *Journal of Advanced Nursing* (November 1998): 28(5):1063–70.

183: *"alcoholism"*: Reported in H. G. Koenig et al., "Religious practices and alcoholism in a southern adult population," *Hospital and Community Psychiatry* (March 1994): 45(3):225–31.

183: *"depressive symptoms"*: Reported in H. G. Koenig et al., "Modeling the cross-sectional relationships between religion, physical health, social support, and depressive symptoms," *American Journal of Geriatric Psychiatry* (Spring 1997): 5(2):131–44.

184: *"Do not conform"*: Romans 12:2.

184: *"Blessed is the man"*: Psalm 1:1–3.

185: *"Encouragement Bible"*: J. E. Tada, D. Dravecky, and J. Dravecky, eds., *NIV Encouragement Bible* (Grand Rapids: Zondervan, 2001).

185: *Lotz*: Anne Graham Lotz, *Daily Light Devotional* (Nashville: Countryman, 1998).

186: *"Several medical studies"*: See, for example, V. Carson and K. Huss, "Prayer—an effective therapeutic and teaching tool," *Journal of Psychiatric Nursing and Mental Health Services* (March 1979): 17(3):34–37.

186: *"One study showed"*: Reported in H. Ayele et al., "Religious activity improves life satisfaction for some physicians and older patients," *Journal of the American Geriatrics Society* (April 1999): 47(4):453–55.

187: *"attitudes were negative"*: Reported in M. V. Mondloch, D. C. Cole, and J. W. Frank, "Does how you do depend on how you think you'll do? A systematic review of the evidence for a relation between patients' recovery expectations and health outcomes," *Canadian Medical Association Journal* (24 July 2001): 165(2):174–79.

187: *"Whatever is true"*: Philippians 4:8–9.

187: *"Unbreakable Bonds"*: Cheryl Meier and Paul Meier, *Unbreakable Bonds: Practicing the Art of Loving and Being Loved* (Grand Rapids: Baker, 2002).

188: *"Families eat less"*: Charles Downey, "Helping Your Child Avoid Obesity"; on the Web at www.scoutingmagazine.org/archives/9901/d-famt.html.

189: *"sitting down together"*: For more on the benefits of shared meals, see "Say 'yes' to family meals"; on the Web at www.extension.iastate.edu/Publications/PM1842.pdf.

189: *"Sharing daily meals"*: Reported in E. Compan et al., "Doing things together: adolescent health and family rituals," *Journal of Epidemiology and Community Health* (February 2002): 56(2):89–94.

189: *"parents were present"*: Reported in Erinn Figg, "Return to the Family Meal. Eating Together Puts Communication Back on Your Menu"; on the Web at www.nsc.org/pubs/fsh/archive/win00/commun.htm.

189: *"Honor your father"*: Exodus 20:12.

190: *"iron sharpens iron"*: Proverbs 27:17; 17:22.

190: *"man of many companions"*: Proverbs 18:24.

190: *"Intimacy is what is needed"*: Minirth and Meier, *Happiness Is a Choice,* 144.

191: *"If an individual"*: Minirth and Meier, *Happiness Is a Choice,* 132.

191: *"There is a kind of"*: Steve Wilson, "Happiness Is an Inside Job"; on the Web at www.stevewilson.com/esteem3.html.

192: *"older people in Japan"*: Reported in N. Krause et al., "Religion, social support, and health among the Japanese elderly," *Journal of Health and Social Behavior* (December 1999): 40(4):405–21.

193: *"We must all wage"*: Jim Rohn, "Overcoming negative thinking"; on the Web at www.foreclosures.com/forecast/ff_oct01/default.asp?topic=great.

Chapter Ten: Nurture Your Hopes and Dreams

196: *"may have life"*: John 10:10.

196: *"believer has an opportunity"*: Frank Minirth, Paul Meier, Richard Meier, and Don Hawkins, *The Healthy Christian Life* (Grand Rapids: Baker, 1988), 25–26.

196: *"I urge you"*: Romans 12:1–2.

197: *"But seek first"*: Matthew 6:33.

197: *"Purpose is not a thing"*: Richard Leider, *The Power of Purpose: Creating Meaning in Your Life and Work* (San Francisco: Berrett-Koehler, 1997), 30.

197: *Bruner*: Kurt Bruner, *The Divine Drama* (Wheaton, Ill.: Tyndale House, 2002).

199: *Peel*: Bill and Kathy Peel, *Discover Your Destiny: Finding the Courage to Follow Your Dreams* (Colorado Springs: NavPress, 1997).

200–201: *"The research suggests"*: Don Ardell, "What Is Wellness?"; on the Web at www.seekwellness.com/WELLNESS/what_is_wellness.htm.

201: *"Another researcher"*: Reported in "Daily Living Tips"; on the Web at www.remicade-ra.com/b_living_with_ra/b4.html.

201: *"a sense of purpose"*: Bonnie Benard, "Fostering Resilience in Children," *ERIC Digest* (August 1995); can be viewed on the Web at www.ed.gov/databases/ERIC_Digests/ed386327.html.

201: *"Passion is doing something"*: Boyd J. Slomoff, "Embrace life: Fulfill your life purpose," *Hawaii Dental Journal* (July–August 2001): 32(4):9.

203: *"Believe deep down"*: Cited in "Inspirational Quotations—2000"; on the Web at http://smiley963.tripod.com/ins2000.html.

203: *"If we all did"*: "Quotations That Inspire"; can be viewed on the Web at http://www.geocities.com/ormead/quotations/quotes.htm.

204: *"a daring adventure"*: "Helen Keller"; can be viewed on the Web at http://www.thinkexist.com/English/Author/x/Author_3057_2.htm.

206: *"Alternative Medicine"*: Dónal O'Mathúna and Walt Larimore, *Alternative Medicine: The Christian Handbook* (Grand Rapids: Zondervan, 2001).

206–7: *"Investigators agree"*: Reported in S. Downing and J. Jura Jr., "Fostering hope in the clinical setting," *Bioethics Forum* (Spring 1999): 15(1):21–24.

207: *"Hope has been shown"*: Reported in J. G. Bruhn, "Therapeutic value of hope," *Southern Medical Journal* (February 1984): 77(2):215–19.

207: *"demoralization"*: Reported in D. W. Kissane, "Demoralisation: its impact on informed consent and medical care," *The Medical Journal of Australia* (November 2001): 175(10):537–39.

207: *"The study concluded"*: Reported in K. F. McFarland et al., "Meaning of illness and health outcomes in type 1 diabetes," *Endocrine Practice* (July–August 2001): 7(4):250–55.

209: *"this simple exercise"*: Based on Gabriel Najera, "Having Trouble Identifying Your True Purpose in Life?"; on the Web at www.todolatino.com/development/tip2.htm.

209: *"can change choice"*: Slomoff, "Embrace life: Fulfill your life purpose."

Chapter Eleven: Be Your Own Health Care Quarterback

211: *"You have the right"*: Isadore Rosenfeld, "Power to the Patient," *Parade Magazine* (24 February 2002): cover.

211: *"medical care is rationed"*: Rosenfeld, "Power to the Patient," 4.

214: *"Knowledge is power"*: Rosenfeld, "Power to the Patient," 5.

218: *"medical errors"*: Medical errors are a major cause of death and injury in America. You can reduce your risk of being a victim of medical error by becoming your own health care quarterback. Check out the United States Agency for Healthcare Research and Quality's twenty tips for reducing your risk via my Website at www.highlyhealthy.net.

220: *"survey of urologic surgeons"*: Reported in F. J. Fowler et al., "Comparison of recommendations by urologists and radiation oncologists for treatment of clinically localized prostate cancer," *Journal of the American Medical Association* (2000): 283(24):3217–22.

221: *"Is any one of you"*: James 5:14.

223: *"The study concluded"*: Reported in "Patient Fact Sheet: 20 Tips to Help Prevent Medical Errors"; on the Web at http://www.ahcpr.gov/consumer/20tips.htm.

228: *"via my Website"*: Turn your Internet browser to www.highlyhealthy.net. Click on this chapter, and then locate and click on this hyperlink.

231: *"work for our good"*: See Romans 8:28.

Chapter Twelve: Team Up with Winning Health Care Providers

236: *Meier*: Paul Meier, *Don't Let Jerks Get the Best of You: Advice for Dealing with Difficult People* (Nashville: Nelson, 1995); Jan Silvious, *Fool-Proofing Your Life: Wisdom for Untangling Your Most Difficult Relationships* (Colorado Springs: WaterBrook, 1998).

239: *"The Bible encourages"*: See 1 Timothy 2:2; Titus 2:2–8.

239: *Hendricks*: Howard and William Hendricks: *As Iron Sharpens Iron: Building Character in a Mentoring Relationship* (Chicago: Moody Press, 1995), 19.

240: *"studies are showing"*: Reported in Harold G. Koenig, Michael E. McCullough, and David B. Larson, *Handbook of Religion and Health* (New York: Oxford Univ. Press, 2000), 104–6, 116–17, 125–26, 151–52, 199–200, 247–49, 313–14, 322, 341, 350–52, 355–57, 368–69.

240: *"one group of researchers"*: Reported in M. M. Paloma and B. F. Pendleton, "Religious domain and general well-being," *Social Indicators Research* (1990): 22:255–76; and "The effects of prayer and prayer experiences on measures of general well-being," *Journal of Psychology and Theology* (1991): 19:71–83.

240: *"cardiologist Robert Byrd"*: Reported in R. C. Byrd, "Positive therapeutic effects of intercessory prayer in a coronary care unit population," *Southern Medical Journal* (1988): 81:826–29.

240: *"intercessory prayer"*: Reported in D. A. Matthews, S. M. Marlowe, and F. S. MacNutt, "Effects of intercessory prayer on patients with rheumatoid arthritis," *Southern Medical Journal* (December 2000): 93(12):1177–86.

240: *"statistically significant"*: Reported in K. Y. Cha, D. P. Wirth, and R. A. Lobo, "Does prayer influence the success of in vitro fertilization embryo transfer? Report of a masked, randomized trial," *Journal of Reproductive*

Medicine (2001): 46(9):781–87.

242: *"The study reported"*: Reported in "Health Technology Case Study 37—Nurse Practitioners, Physician Assistants, and Certified Nurse-Midwives: A Policy Analysis" (Washington D.C.: Office of Technology Assessment, December 1986).

242: *New Life Clinics*: You can reach the Meier New Life Clinics at 1-800-NEW-LIFE, on the Web at www.newlife.com/Meier_Clinics/meier_clinics.htm.

244: *Order of St. Luke*: The International Order of St. Luke the Physician is a Christian healing ministry and fellowship of (1) professional people in all phases of medical work; (2) clergy in the ministry of the Roman, Orthodox, Anglican, and Protestant churches; and (3) laypeople from all walks of life who believe that the healing ministry of Jesus Christ belongs in the church today. The order is the outgrowth of the Fellowship of Saint Luke, begun in 1932 by the late John Gayner Banks, S.T.D., priest of the Episcopal Church, and his wife, Ethel Tulloch Banks.

244: *Stephen Ministry*: For over twenty-five years, Stephen Ministries has been serving thousands of congregations from more than one hundred denominations with biblical, Christ-centered training and resources for one-to-one lay care giving, small groups, and spiritual growth and healing.

244: *"via my Website"*: Turn your Internet browser to www.highlyhealthy.net. Click on this chapter, and then locate and click on this hyperlink.

245: *"No such condition"*: S. Barrett, "Chiropractic's Elusive 'Subluxation'"; on the Web at www.quackwatch.com/01QuackeryRelatedTopics/chirosub.html.

245: *"Spinal manipulation"*: Samuel Homola, "What a Rational Chiropractor Can Do for You"; on the Web at www.chirobase.org/07Strategy/goodchiro.html [article adapted from *Inside Chiropractic: A Patient's Guide* (New York: Prometheus, 1999)].

246: *"Alternative Medicine"*: Dónal O'Mathúna and Walt Larimore, *Alternative Medicine: The Christian Handbook* (Grand Rapids: Zondervan, 2001).

248: *"you can access"*: Turn your Internet browser to www.highlyhealthy.net. Click on this chapter, and then locate and click on this hyperlink.

249: *McCall*: See Timothy B. McCall, *Examining Your Doctor: A Patient's Guide to Avoiding Harmful Medical Care* (New York: Birch Lane Press, 1995).

249: *"via my Website"*: Turn your Internet browser to www.highlyhealthy.net. Click on this chapter, and then locate and click on this hyperlink.

251: *"selecting your spouse"*: See Isadore Rosenfeld, *Power to the Patient: The Treatments to Insist On When You're Sick* (New York: Warner, 2002).

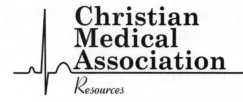

Christian
Medical
Association
Resources

Medically reliable . . . biblically sound. That's the rock-solid promise of this series offered by Zondervan in partnership with the Christian Medical Association. Each book in this series is not only written by fully credentialed, experienced doctors but is also fully reviewed by an objective board of qualified doctors to ensure its reliability. Because when your health is at stake, you can't settle for anything less than the whole and accurate truth.

Integrating your faith and health can improve your physical well-being and even extend your life, as you gain insights into the interconnection of health and faith—a relationship largely overlooked by secular science. Benefit from the cutting-edge knowledge of respected medical experts as they help you make health care decisions consistent with your beliefs. Their sound biblical analysis of emerging treatments and technologies equips you to protect yourself from seemingly harmless—yet spiritually, ethically, or medically unsound—options and then to make the healthiest choices possible.

Through this series, you can draw from both the knowledge of science and the wisdom of God's Word in addressing your medical ethics decisions and in meeting your health care needs.

Founded in 1931, the Christian Medical Association helps thousands of doctors minister to their patients by imitating the Great Physician, Jesus Christ. Christian Medical Association members provide a Christian voice on medical ethics to policy makers and the media, minister to needy patients on medical missions around the world, evangelize and disciple students on more than 90 percent of the nation's medical school campuses, and provide educational and inspirational resources to the church.

To learn more about Christian Medical Association ministries and resources on health care and ethical issues, browse the website (www.christian medicalassociation.org) or call toll-free at 1-888-231-2637.

"Dear friend, I pray that you may enjoy good health and that all may
go well with you, even as your soul is getting along well" (3 John 2).

God's Design for the Highly Healthy Child

*Walt Larimore, M.D.,
with Stephen and Amanda Sorenson*

You want the best for your child, especially when it comes to his or her health. You can cut through popular misconceptions and discover the surprising and proven connections between a child's physical, emotional, relational, and spiritual health.

No matter what the obstacles, your child can become more highly healthy. *God's Design for the Highly Healthy Child* will teach you, in very practical ways, how to assess your child's health, fix the "spoke" that's broke, and follow advice that can make a difference in your child's health immediately.

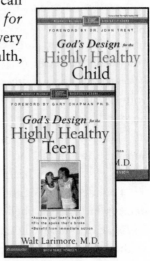

God's Design for the Highly Healthy Teen

*Walt Larimore, M.D.,
with Mike Yorkey*

Good news! An on-call, day or night health consultant for parents—now available for you during those critical (and often scary) teen years. Dr. Walt Larimore is on call, and he's applying his wisdom to your teen's health.

God's Design for the Highly Healthy Teen will help you assess your teen's health, zero in where your teen's health is out of balance, and follow practical, achievable advice that can result in positive changes in your teen's life—and in the process, you'll become a more highly healthy parent.

Softcover: 0-310-26279-8

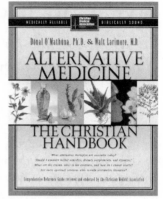
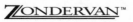

Bryson City Tales

Stories of a Doctor's First Year
of Practice in the Smoky Mountains

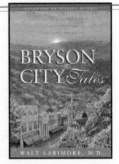

The little mountain hamlet of Bryson City, North Carolina, offers more than dazzling vistas. For Walt Larimore, a young "flatlander" physician setting up his first practice, the town presents its peculiar challenges as well. Sharing the joys, heartaches, frustrations, and rewards of rural mountain medical practice, *Bryson City Tales* is a tender and insightful chronicle of a young man's rite of passage from medical student to family physician. Laughter and adventure await you in these pages, and lessons learned from the strengths, foibles, and simple faith of Bryson City's unforgettable residents.

Softcover: 0-310-25670-4

Bryson City Seasons

More Tales of a Doctor's Practice
in the Smoky Mountains

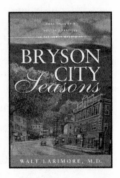

Dr. Walt Larimore whisks you along on a journey through the seasons of another year in Bryson City. On the way you'll encounter crusty mountain men, warmhearted townspeople, peppery medical personalities, and the hallmarks of a more wholesome way of life. Dr. Larimore's vibrant slices of small-town living will capture your imagination and inspire your heart. Lit with love, humor, glowing faith, and the warmth of family and friendships, *Bryson City Seasons* is a celebration of this richly textured miracle called life.

Hardcover: 0-310-25287-3

Pick up a copy at your favorite bookstore today!

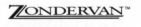

Resources by Dr. Walt Larimore

Bryson City Seasons

Bryson City Tales

Alternative Medicine: The Christian Handbook
   (coauthored with Dónal O'Mathúna)

God's Design for the Highly Healthy Person
   (with Traci Mullins)

God's Design for the Highly Healthy Child
   (with Stephen and Amanda Sorenson)

God's Design for the Highly Healthy Teen
   (with Mike Yorkey)

Why ADHD Doesn't Mean Disaster
   (coauthored with Dennis Swanberg and Diane Passno)

Lintball Leo's Not-So-Stupid Questions About Your Body
   (with John Riddle, illustrated by Mike Phillips)

Going Public with Your Faith: Becoming a Spiritual Influence at Work
   (coauthored with William Carr Peel)

Going Public with Your Faith: Becoming a Spiritual Influence at Work
   audio
      (coauthored with William Carr Peel)

Going Public with Your Faith: Becoming a Spiritual Influence at Work
   Zondervan*Groupware*™ curriculum
      (coauthored with William Carr Peel, with Stephen
         and Amanda Sorenson)

Praise for *God's Design for the Highly Healthy Person*

Walt Larimore, M.D., has been considered for many years to be "America's Doctor" because of his national television and radio call-in programs. Walt is a brilliant and loving physician who does his research and has immense common sense as well. I personally found *God's Design for the Highly Healthy Person* extremely helpful and practical. I'm convinced that anyone who reads it and applies it will greatly enhance his or her own quality of life and be given tools to benefit the lives of those they love.

—PAUL MEIER, M.D.
Founder, Meier New Life Clinics

This is the best book on healthy living I've ever read. Its holistic yet practical approach will transform your life.

—DAVID STEVENS, M.D., M.A. (Ethics)
Executive director, Christian Medical & Dental Associations

There are so many people in our society who feel sick because they lack balance and peace in their lives. Dr. Walt offers advice to show all of us the way back to highly healthy living.

—BRUCE BAGLEY, M.D.
Past president, American Academy of Family Physicians

Packed with valuable insights from a career in family medicine, *God's Design for the Highly Healthy Person* brings a refreshing and important simplicity to the complex world of health for the layperson. Dr. Larimore's passion and advocacy for prevention and wholeness make this book an excellent resource.

—ROBERT G. BROOKS, M.D.
Professor of family medicine,
Florida State University College of Medicine

God's Design for the Highly Healthy Person is an easy-to-read map for a "road trip" with a physician-guide who draws on years of clinical experience. Finding balance and symmetry to make the wheels of life run smoothly, Dr. Larimore encourages the reader to make proactive lifestyle choices in the critical areas of physical, relational, emotional, and spiritual well-being. This practical guide involves the reader with exercises, surveys, and soul-searching questions to point the way beyond disease prevention and on to total wellness.

—WILLIAM R. CUTRER, M.D.
Professor of Christian ministry,
The Southern Baptist Theological Seminary